Promoting Safe and Effective Genetic Testing in the United States

Final Report of the Task Force on Genetic Testing

EDITED BY

Neil A. Holtzman, M.D., M.P.H.

AND

Michael S. Watson, Ph.D.

THE JOHNS HOPKINS UNIVERSITY PRESS

Baltimore and London

New material © 1998 The Johns Hopkins University Press
All rights reserved. Published 1998
Printed in the United States of America on acid-free paper
2   4   6   8   9   7   5   3   1

The Johns Hopkins University Press
2715 North Charles Street, Baltimore, Maryland 21218-4363
The Johns Hopkins Press Ltd., London
www.press.jhu.edu

Library of Congress Cataloging-in-Publication Data will be found at the end of this book.
A catalog record for this book is available from the British Library.

ISBN 0-8018-5952-2   ISBN 0-8018-5972-7 (pbk.)

Contents

6. SUMMARY AND CONCLUSIONS   87

APPENDICES

Preface to the Johns Hopkins University Press Edition

The Task Force on Genetic Testing was an official government advisory group reporting to the National Advisory Council for Human Genome Research of the National Human Genome Research Institute (NHGRI), the National Institutes of Health. The final report of the Task Force was first released in September of 1997 in a limited edition distributed by NHGRI. A few weeks later, the report (including appendices) was made available on the World-Wide Web at http://www.nhgri.nih.gov/ELSI/TFGT_final/, where it is still accessible. Those who wish to see two preliminary working documents of the Task Force, the Interim Principles and Proposed Recommendations and the full, final report, can view them at http://www.med.jhu.edu/tfgtelsi. The Proposed Recommendations were also published in the *Federal Register* (1997;62:4539–4547). Although the Task Force incorporated most of the Interim Principles into its final report, it significantly revised the Proposed Recommendations, largely in response to public comments. Neither the Interim Principles nor the Proposed Recommendations represent the final policies of the Task Force.

To make the final report more widely accessible, the Task Force sought and obtained agreement with the Johns Hopkins University Press to publish this edition at a low price. Neither the Task Force nor any other organization or individual will receive royalties from the sale of this edition.

First editions often contain words or phrases that could be improved. The Task Force calls the reader's attention to three changes in this edition. First, in the definition of genetic tests (pp. xi and 6), the word *inherited* has been substituted for *heritable*. The latter is generally viewed as a statistical concept, whereas the Task Force means actual, identifiable mutations transmitted from one generation to the next. Second, in "Types of problems encountered in predictive genetic testing" (Box, p. 23), the Task Force has provided examples that more clearly indicate problems of analytical validity than those originally given in (b) and (c) under the first bullet. Third, to maintain consistency, the Task Force has substituted the word *request* for *require* in its recommendation on provider competence (pp. xxii, 67, and 87). The recommendation now is consistent with the statement (p. 69) that "the Task Force does not favor *requiring* organizations to establish competence requirements (emphasis added)." In Appendix 2, the "Background" has been expanded to explain more clearly the origins of the Task Force's letter to FDA, which constitutes the main body of Appendix 2. Several small changes, most stylistic, have been made by the author of Appendix 5. We have also corrected typographical errors and updated references for work that has been published since the original report. In addition, an index of subjects and authorities cited in the text has been added, and the Table of Contents streamlined.

The Task Force is pleased with the recognition given to its work. Secretary of Health and Human Services Donna Shalala has maintained an interest in the work of the Task Force throughout its deliberations and is considering the recommendations in the final report. In addition, the Clinical Laboratory Improvement Advisory Committee has created a genetics subcommittee to consider the recommendations to ensure the quality of laboratories performing genetic tests. Issues relating to the role of Institutional Review Boards are also being considered by President Clinton's National Bioethics Advisory Committee. Thus it seems likely that this report, which now can be widely read, will not languish on bookshelves.

Acknowledgments

The work of the Task Force was accomplished with the help of many others. **Joshua Brown** served as staff attorney for the Task Force from April 1995 to May 1996. Mr. Brown prepared very helpful briefing materials and presentations for the Task Force on laws and regulations relating to genetic testing, coordinated Task Force committee meetings, and assisted in the formulation of Task Force principles and recommendations. After Mr. Brown's departure, **Emily Koscianski** and **Andrew Siegel** continued legislative and regulatory analysis and the drafting of proposed recommendations on a part-time basis until April 1997. Dr. Siegel, a Greenwall Fellow, was particularly helpful in framing issues related to institutional review boards. **Jodi Goldstein, Taria Herz, Kathleen Lester, Amanda Merwin,** and **Michele Schoonmaker,** at the time graduate students at the Johns Hopkins School of Hygiene and Public Health (Goldstein and Lester in the joint Hopkins-Georgetown University program in law, ethics, and health), also prepared very useful background papers. **Jane Fullarton**'s familiarity with the Department of Health and Human Services proved extremely valuable in preparing the Task Force's proposed recommendations.

At the Genetics and Public Policy Studies unit at the Johns Hopkins Medical Institutions, where much of the work was done, **Sharon Ennis** coordinated administrative tasks and **Robbin Wingfield-Street** maintained mailing lists and assembled briefing materials for the Task Force. Over the more than 2-year life of the Task Force, **Tascon** was responsible for scheduling and arranging meetings (including travel of Task Force members), final mailings, publication of the report, and overall administration. We wish to thank, particularly, **Rose Salton, Cindy Elliott-Amadon,** and **Nancy Shapiro.**

The appendices to the report were edited by **Alice Lium,** and the main body of the report by **Barbara Cobb. Cindy James,** a graduate student in genetic counseling and human genetics, checked references and analyzed trends in genetic discoveries and resources.

Support for the Task Force was generously provided by the National Human Genome Research Institute (NHGRI). The Task Force is grateful for the personal interest **Francis Collins, Director of NHGRI,** took in its work and for his very helpful input.

Finally, every voting and liaison member of the Task Force played an active role in the development of the Task Force's principles and recommendations, and the preparation of the report. **Patricia Murphy** generously agreed to help in the writing of Chapter 3. **Carlyn Collins** of the Centers for Disease Control and Prevention, **Kate Kremann** of the Health Care Financing Administration, and **Freda Yoder** of the Food and Drug Administration attended many Task Force meetings, reviewed briefing materials and drafts, and made many helpful suggestions.

Members of the

Task Force on Genetic Testing

<u>Voting Members and the Organizations They Represented:</u>

Neil A. Holtzman, M.D., M.P.H., <u>Chair</u>
National Institutes of Health–Department of Energy Working Group on Ethical, Legal, and
    Social Implications of Human Genome Research (ELSI Working Group)

Michael S. Watson, Ph.D., FACMG, <u>Co-Chair</u>
American College of Medical Genetics

Patricia A. Barr
National Breast Cancer Coalition

David R. Cox, M.D., Ph.D.*
ELSI Working Group

Jessica G. Davis, M.D.
Council of Regional Networks for Genetic Services

Stephen I. Goodman, M.D., M.Sc.
American Society of Human Genetics

Wayne W. Grody, M.D., Ph.D.
College of American Pathologists

Arthur L. Levin, M.D.
Alliance for Managed Competition

J. Alexander Lowden, M.D., Ph.D.
Health Insurance Association of America

Patricia D. Murphy, Ph.D., FACMG
OncorMed

Patricia J. Numann, M.D.
American Medical Association

Victoria O. Odesina, R.N., Sc.M., M.S.
Alliance of Genetic Support Groups

Nancy Press, Ph.D.
ELSI Working Group

Katherine A. Schneider, M.P.H.
National Society of Genetic Counselors

David B. Singer
Biotechnology Industry Organization (BIO)
Elliott Hillback was BIO alternate representative when Mr. Singer could not attend.

Government Liaison (Non-voting) Members:

Steven Gutman, M.D.
Food and Drug Administration

Muin J. Khoury, M.D., Ph.D.
Centers for Disease Control and Prevention

David Lanier, M.D.
Agency for Health Care Policy and Research
Peter Bouxsein, M.D. represented the Agency until September 1996.

Linda R. Lebovic
Health Care Financing Administration

Jane S. Lin-Fu, M.D.
Health Resources and Services Administration

The work of the Task Force was supported by the National Institutes of Health.

---

*Dr. Cox does not condone any changes made to the final Task Force report and does not wish his name to be associated with this edition of the report.

EXECUTIVE SUMMARY

The rapid pace of discovery of genetic factors in disease has improved our ability to predict risks of disease in asymptomatic individuals. We have learned how to prevent the manifestations of a few of these diseases and treat some others. Gene therapy is being actively investigated.

Despite remarkable progress much remains unknown about the risks and benefits of genetic testing.

- No effective interventions are yet available to improve the outcome of most inherited diseases.
- Negative (normal) test results might not rule out future occurrence of disease.
- Positive test results might not mean the disease will inevitably develop.

It is primarily in the context of their unknown potential risks and benefits that the Task Force considers genetic tests.

Origin and Work of the Task Force

The Task Force was created by the National Institutes of Health (NIH)-Department of Energy (DOE) Working Group on Ethical, Legal, and Social Implications (ELSI) of Human Genome Research to review genetic testing in the United States and make recommendations to ensure the development of safe and effective genetic tests. The Task Force has defined safety and effectiveness to encompass not only the validity and utility of genetic tests, but their delivery in laboratories of assured quality, and their appropriate use by health care providers and consumers.

The Working Group invited organizations with a stake in genetic testing to submit nominations from which it selected members of the Task Force. In addition, the Working Group invited five agencies in the Department of Health and Human Services (HHS) to send nonvoting liaison members to the Task Force. Principles and recommendations of the Task Force appear in **bold-faced type.**

Definition of Genetic Tests

Genetic test--The analysis of human DNA, RNA, chromosomes, proteins, and certain metabolites in order to detect inherited disease-related genotypes, mutations, phenotypes, or karyotypes for clinical purposes. Such purposes include predicting risk of disease, identifying carriers, and establishing prenatal and clinical diagnosis or prognosis. Prenatal, newborn and carrier screening, as well as testing in high risk families, are included. Tests for metabolites are covered only when they are undertaken with high probability that an excess or deficiency of the metabolite indicates the presence of inherited mutations in single genes. Tests conducted purely for research are excluded from the definition, as are tests for somatic (as opposed to inherited) mutations, and testing for forensic purposes.

The Task Force is primarily concerned about predictive uses of genetic tests performed in healthy or apparently healthy people. Predictive test results do not necessarily mean that the disease will inevitably occur or remain absent; they replace the individual's prior risks based on population data or family history with risks based on genotype. Some, but not all, predictive genetic testing falls under the rubric "genetic screening," a search in a <u>population</u> for persons possessing certain genotypes.

<u>The Need for Recommendations</u>

For the most part, genetic testing in the United States has developed successfully, providing options for avoiding, preventing, and treating inherited disorders. However, problems arise as a result of current practices.

- Sometimes, genetic tests are introduced before they have been demonstrated to be safe, effective, and useful (see chapter 2 and appendices 5 and 6).
- There is no assurance that every laboratory performing genetic tests for clinical purposes meets high standards (see chapter 3).
- Often, the informational materials distributed by academic and commercial genetic testing laboratories do not provide sufficient information to fill in the gaps in providers' and patients' understanding of genetic tests (see appendix 4).
- In the next few years, a greater burden for offering genetic testing will fall on providers who have little formal training or experience in genetics.

In this report, the Task Force does not recommend policies for specific tests but suggests a framework for ensuring that new tests meet criteria for safety and effectiveness before they are unconditionally released, thereby reducing the likelihood of premature clinical use. **The focus of the Task Force on potential problems in no way is intended to detract from the benefits of genetic testing. Its overriding goal is to recommend policies that will reduce the likelihood of damaging effects so the benefits of testing can be fully realized undiluted by harm.**

<u>Need for an Advisory Committee on Genetic Testing</u>

The Task Force calls on the Secretary of Health and Human Services (HHS) to establish an advisory committee on genetic testing in the Office of the Secretary. Members of the committee should represent the stakeholders in genetic testing, including professional societies (general medicine, genetics, pathology, genetic counseling), the biotechnology industry, consumers, and insurers, as well as other interested parties. The various HHS agencies with activities related to the development and delivery of genetic tests should send nonvoting representatives to the advisory committee, which can also coordinate the relevant activities of these agencies and private organizations. The Task Force leaves it to the Secretary to determine the relationship of this advisory committee to others that may be created in the broader area of genetics and public policy, of which genetic testing is only one part.

The committee would advise the Secretary on implementation of recommendations made by the Task Force in this report to ensure that (a) the introduction of new genetic tests into clinical use is based on evidence of their analytical and clinical validity, and utility to those tested; (b) all stages of the genetic testing process in clinical laboratories meet quality standards; (c) health providers who offer and order genetic tests have sufficient competence in genetics and genetic testing to protect the well-being of their patients; and (d) there be continued and expanded availability of tests for rare genetic diseases.

The Task Force recognizes the widely inclusive nature of genetic tests. It is therefore essential that the advisory committee recommend policies for the Secretary's consideration by which agencies and organizations implementing recommendations can determine those genetic tests that need stringent scrutiny. Stringent scrutiny is indicated when a test has the ability to predict future inherited disease in healthy or apparently healthy people, is likely to be used for that purpose, and when no confirmatory test is available. The advisory committee or its designate should define additional indications.

In order to carry out its functions, the advisory committee should have its own staff and budget.

The Task Force further recommends that the Secretary review the accomplishments of the advisory committee on genetic testing after 2 full years of operation and determine whether it should continue to operate.

Overarching Principles

In making recommendations on safety and effectiveness, the Task Force concentrated on test validity and utility, laboratory quality, and provider competence. It recognizes, however, that other issues impinge on testing, and problems may arise from testing. Regarding these issues, the Task Force endorses the following principles.

Informed Consent. The Task Force strongly advocates written informed consent. The failure of the Task Force to comment on informed consent for other uses does not imply that it should not be obtained.

Test Development. Informed consent for any validation study must be obtained whenever the specimen can be linked to the subject from which it came.

Testing in Clinical Practice. (1) It is unacceptable to coerce or intimidate individuals or families regarding their decision about predictive genetic testing. Respect for personal autonomy is paramount. People being offered testing must understand that testing is voluntary. Their informed consent should be obtained. Whatever decision they make, their care should not be jeopardized.

(2) Prior to the initiation of predictive testing in clinical practice, health care providers must describe the features of the genetic test, including potential consequences, to potential test recipients.

Newborn Screening. (1) If informed consent is waived for a newborn screening test, the analytical and clinical validity and clinical utility of the test must be established, and parents must be provided with sufficient information to understand the reasons for screening. By clinical utility, the Task Force means that interventions to improve the outcome of the infant identified by screening have been proven to be safe and effective.

(2) For those disorders for which newborn screening is available but the tests have not been validated or shown to have clinical utility, written parental consent is required prior to testing.

Prenatal and Carrier Testing. Respect for an individual's/couples' beliefs and values concerning tests undertaken for assisting reproductive decisions is of paramount importance and can best be maintained by a nondirective stance. One way of ensuring that a non-directive stance is taken and that parents' decisions are autonomous, is through requiring informed consent.

Testing of Children. **Genetic testing of children for adult onset diseases should not be undertaken unless direct medical benefit will accrue to the child and this benefit would be lost by waiting until the child has reached adulthood.**

Confidentiality. Protecting the confidentiality of information is essential for all uses of genetic tests. **(1) Results should be released only to those individuals for whom the test recipient has given consent for information release. Means of transmitting information should be chosen to minimize the likelihood that results will become available to unauthorized persons or organizations. Under no circumstances should results with identifiers be provided to any outside parties, including employers, insurers, or government agencies, without the test recipient's written consent.**

(2) Health care providers have an obligation to the person being tested not to inform other family members without the permission of the person tested, except in extreme circumstances.

Discrimination. **No individual should be subjected to unfair discrimination by a third party on the basis of having had a genetic test or receiving an abnormal genetic test result.** Third parties include insurers, employers, and educational and other institutions that routinely inquire about the health of applicants for services or positions.

Consumer Involvement in Policy Making. Although other stakeholders are concerned about protecting consumers, they cannot always provide the perspective brought by consumers themselves, the end users of genetic testing. **Consumers should be involved in policy (but not necessarily in technical) decisions regarding the adoption, introduction, and use of new, predictive genetic tests.**

ENSURING THE SAFETY AND EFFECTIVENESS OF NEW GENETIC TESTS

Providers and consumers cannot make a fully-informed decision about whether or not to use genetic tests unless their benefits and risks have been assessed. Although extensive use has eventually proved most tests to be of benefit, a few eventually proved unhelpful and were discarded. In the meantime, people were wrongly classified as at-risk and subjected to treatments that, in their case, proved unnecessary or sometimes harmful. Others, who could have benefited from treatment were classified as "normal" and denied treatment. The Task Force strongly recommends that the following criteria be satisfied.

(1) **The genotypes to be detected by a genetic test must be shown by scientifically valid methods to be associated with the occurrence of a disease. The observations must be independently replicated and subject to peer review.**

(2) **Analytical sensitivity and specificity of a genetic test must be determined before it is made available in clinical practice.**

(3) **Data to establish the clinical validity of genetic tests (clinical sensitivity, specificity, and predictive value) must be collected under investigative protocols. In clinical validation,**

the study sample must be drawn from a group of subjects representative of the population for whom the test is intended. Formal validation for each intended use of a genetic test is needed.

(4) Before a genetic test can be generally accepted in clinical practice, data must be collected to demonstrate the benefits and risks that accrue from both positive and negative results.

Ensuring Compliance with Criteria for Safety and Effectiveness

Because of the length of time it can take to establish the appropriateness of a test for clinical use, it is all the more important to ensure the collection of data on safety and effectiveness in the course of test development. At present, no government policy requires the collection of data on clinical validity and utility for all predictive genetic tests under development.

Considering the structures for external review of research in the U.S. today, the Task Force is of the opinion that institutional review boards (IRBs) are the most appropriate organizations to consider whether the scientific merit of protocols for the development of genetic tests warrants the risk to subjects participating in the research.

Protocols for the development of genetic tests that can be used predictively must receive the approval of an institutional review board (IRB) when subject identifiers are retained and when the intention is to make the test readily available for clinical use, i.e., to market the test. IRB review should consider the adequacy of the protocol for: (a) the protection of human subjects involved in the study, and (b) the collection of data on analytic and clinical validity, and data on the test's utility for individuals who are tested.

Tests under development must be conducted in laboratories certified under the Clinical Laboratory Improvement Amendments (CLIA) if the results will be reported to patients or their providers.

Health department laboratories or other public agencies developing new genetic tests that satisfy these conditions must also submit protocols to properly constituted IRBs.

The Task Force recommends that the Office of Protection of Human Subjects from Research Risks (OPRR) develop guidelines to assist IRBs in reviewing genetic testing protocols. The proposed Secretary's Advisory Committee should work with OPRR to accomplish this task. In developing guidelines for IRBs, OPRR should focus first on tests under development that require stringent scrutiny. **The proposed Secretary's Advisory Committee or its designate, in cooperation with OPRR, should establish criteria for stringent scrutiny.**

Conflict of Interest. **The Task Force recommends strenuous efforts by all IRBs (commercial and academic) to avoid conflicts of interest, or the appearance of conflicts of interest, when reviewing specific protocols for genetic testing. OPRR should consider more stringent standards for all types of IRBs for avoiding conflict of interest situations.**

Enforcement. **Testing organizations should comply voluntarily with obtaining IRB approval of genetic test protocols.** Other options the Task Force considered for enforcing the requirement for IRB approval included that: (1) the FDA use its authority to require all test developers to submit protocols to IRBs, (2) third-party payers refuse to reimburse for a genetic test unless the developer can show that it conducted validation/utility studies under an IRB-approved protocol, (3) clinical laboratory surveyors (see chapter 3) confirm that laboratories have received IRB approval of the new genetic tests that they developed, and (4) Congress enact legislation requiring submission of all research protocols, regardless of support, to an IRB.

Data Collection. To expedite data collection, collaborative efforts will often be needed. **OPRR, with input from the proposed Secretary's Advisory Committee on genetic testing, should streamline the requirements for IRB review of multicenter collaborative protocols for genetic test development in order to reduce costs and get the studies quickly underway.**

The Task Force calls on Federal agencies, particularly NIH and the Centers for Disease Control and Prevention (CDC) to support consortia and other collaborative efforts to facilitate collection of data on the safety and effectiveness of new genetic tests. CDC should play a coordinating role in data gathering and should be allocated sufficient funds for this purpose. In sharing or pooling of data, confidentiality of the subject source of the data must be strictly maintained.

The Need for Post-market Surveillance. **The Task Force recognizes that assessing the validity and utility of some genetic tests will take a long time. When preliminary data indicate a test is likely to have validity and utility, the test should be approved for marketing (see below) but developers must continue to collect data until more definitive answers are obtained.** Options for encouraging collection of the requisite data include the following:

(1) Voluntary collection of data by developers after their tests enter clinical use.

(2) Reimbursement for, or coverage of, tests by third party payers during investigative stages in which data are being collected.

(3) Conditional premarket approval by the FDA of genetic test kits. In return for conditional approval, developers could include a profit markup in the price while they continue to collect data.

Evidence-based Entry of New Genetic Tests into Clinical Practice

Test developers must submit their validation and clinical utility data to internal as well as independent external review. In addition, test developers should provide information to professional organizations in order to permit informed decisions about routine use. The Task Force recognizes that not all new genetic tests are in need of such review. **The proposed Secretary's Advisory Committee should suggest criteria for external review, and recommend means of ensuring that review of tests requiring stringent scrutiny will take place.** To accomplish the latter, the cooperation of various government and nongovernment groups to conduct reviews must be secured, as well as funds to support the reviews. A wide range of stakeholders should participate in reviews.

Local Review. **The Task Force strongly suggests that any organization in which tests are developed conduct a structured review of the analytic and clinical validity and utility of new genetic tests before marketing them or otherwise making them available for clinical use. This structured review should be conducted by those not actually involved in developing the test and collecting the data.** Some medical centers have standing committees that review tests proposed to be offered in the institution's clinical laboratories that could serve this function. For commercial organizations, a unit within the company, but independent of the laboratory that is actually developing the test, should review the data.

National Review. Current legal requirements that genetic tests be reviewed prior to their clinical use apply only to tests marketed as kits, which require premarket approval by FDA. **To**

improve FDA perspectives on genetic testing and related issues, the Task Force recommends that FDA bring together consultants on genetic testing either from existing panels or by constructing a new panel to provide guidance to FDA on genetic testing devices with single or multiple intended uses.

Although no other legally-required mechanisms currently exist, other reviews can have a profound influence on providers' decisions to use, or not use, new medical technologies. Examples are: statements of professional societies, consensus development panels, and ratings by the U.S. Preventive Services Task Force. The decision of health insurers on whether a specific genetic test will be included in their benefits or reimbursement packages can also influence use and will be based on the insurers' own reviews or other external reviews.

ENSURING THE QUALITY OF LABORATORIES PERFORMING GENETIC TESTS

Although laboratories performing chromosomal, biochemical, and/or DNA-based tests for genetic diseases must comply with general regulations under the Clinical Laboratory Improvement Amendments of 1988 (CLIA), current requirements under CLIA are inadequate to ensure the overall quality of genetic testing because they are not specifically designed for any genetic tests except cytogenetic tests. Most laboratories performing genetic tests voluntarily participate in quality programs addressed specifically to genetic tests, but they are not required to do so. Consequently, providers and consumers have no assurance that every laboratory performs adequately.

Principles for Laboratories Adopting New Genetic Tests

No clinical laboratory should offer a genetic test whose clinical validity has not been established, unless it is collecting data on clinical validity under either an IRB-approved protocol or conditional premarket approval agreement with FDA (one of the options presented in chapter 2. The service laboratory should justify and document the basis of decisions to put new tests into service. Regardless of where the test to be adopted was developed, **clinical laboratory directors are responsible for ensuring the analytic validity of each genetic test their laboratory intends to offer before they make the test available for use in clinical practice (outside of an investigative protocol).**

Before routinely offering genetic tests that have been clinically validated, a laboratory must conduct a pilot phase in which it verifies that all steps in the testing process are operating appropriately. If the pilot study reveals that the laboratory is not as competent as other laboratories in performing the test, or the test does not detect as many people with the genetic alteration as anticipated, the laboratory should not proceed to report patient-specific results without attempting to rectify the problems.

Requirements Under CLIA

The stringency of CLIA requirements depends on the complexity level and specialty to which tests are assigned.

Complexity Ratings. CDC assigns a complexity level to a test according to predetermined criteria. Laboratories performing high complexity tests have more stringent personnel and quality-control requirements. Despite multiple uses, a test method gets only one rating. **The Task Force recommends that tests that can be used for purposes of predicting future disease be given a rating of high complexity.**

CLIA Specialties. Laboratories can perform tests only in specialties for which they are certified. Although there is a cytogenetics specialty, there is no genetics specialty. **The Task Force welcomes the intention of CDC to create a genetics subcommittee of the Clinical Laboratory Improvement Advisory Committee (CLIAC), which advises on policies under CLIA. The Task Force urges this subcommittee to consider the creation of a specialty of genetics that would encompass all predictive genetic tests that satisfy criteria for stringent scrutiny. If a specialty of genetics is not feasible, the subcommittee should consider a specialty or subspecialty of molecular genetics for DNA/RNA-based tests. In the latter case, it must then address how to ensure the quality of laboratories performing nonDNA/RNA genetic tests. The subcommittee should also consider assigning tests that have widely different uses to more than one specialty.**

Laboratory Personnel. Personnel requirements under CLIA, particularly at the level of laboratory director, depend on the specialty and complexity categories to which tests or analytes are assigned. Without a genetics specialty, genetic tests fall into other specialties for which requiring special training in genetics would be superfluous. **The Task Force recommends that, for laboratories performing high complexity tests in the proposed specialty of molecular genetics, as well as in biochemical genetics and cytogenetics, personnel serving as directors or technical supervisors must have formal training in human and medical genetics, as documented by holding certification from an organization that assesses knowledge of human and medical genetics as part of its certification process, such as the American Board of Medical Genetics. Training programs for laboratory technicians/technologists need more human and medical genetics content than are currently available in the U.S.**

Monitoring Laboratory Performance

Because laboratories provide services to providers and patients in many states it is clearly more desirable to have a rigorous Federal standard for certification or accreditation than fifty different State standards. Moreover, interstate genetic testing is unavoidable when only one or a few laboratories in the country provide tests. **A national accreditation program for laboratories performing genetic tests, which includes proficiency testing and onsite inspection, is needed to promote standardization across the country.** Such an accreditation program can occur more readily if a genetics specialty were established under CLIA. **Until such time as a genetics specialty is established under CLIA, laboratories performing DNA/RNA-based tests for predictive purposes should choose to voluntarily participate in the College of American Pathologists' (CAP) molecular pathology program, including the CAP/American College of Medical Genetics (ACMG) molecular genetics proficiency testing program.** Laboratories performing genetic tests on analytes not covered in the CAP/ACMG program, such as Tay-Sachs carrier screening and newborn screening, should participate in the available proficiency programs.

Proficiency Testing (PT). Under CLIA, every laboratory performing moderate or high complexity tests is required to enroll in PT programs recognized by HCFA. Any laboratory that fails a proficiency test must take corrective action.

So far, the Department of Health and Human Services has not approved proficiency testing programs for genetic tests because such tests do not measure regulated analytes for PT purposes. Nevertheless, under CLIA, laboratories must establish the accuracy and reliability of a test by methods of their own choosing. This can include participation in one of the voluntary PT programs. As these programs have not been approved by CLIA, no laboratory is obliged to use them and can establish accuracy and reliability by another method, although it must make the data available for onsite inspection under CLIA (see below).

Participation in well-established proficiency testing programs for genetic tests must be required under CLIA once a genetics specialty is established. When no relevant proficiency testing programs exist, laboratories must, whenever possible, participate in inter-laboratory comparison programs and help develop them if none exist in their particular area of testing.

Proficiency testing programs should be broadly based since the number of genetic disorders is very large and the analytical approaches to testing are numerous.

Onsite Inspection. All CLIA-certified laboratories are routinely inspected on a two-year survey cycle by (1) HCFA regional offices and State agencies, (2) private non-profit organizations to which HCFA has given "deemed" status in recognition of their ability to provide reasonable assurance that the laboratories they accredit meet the conditions required by Federal law, or (3) State-exempt licensure programs.

CAP has deemed status to conduct inspections in several specialties, but since genetics is not a specialty under CLIA, the CAP program does not have deemed status in genetics. In the CAP genetics program, laboratories who voluntarily participate in the program are inspected.

Making Laboratory Performance Assessments Public

Publishing the names of laboratories performing satisfactorily would advise users that labs not appearing on the list have either not submitted to external review or have not performed adequately. HCFA annually publishes a list ("Laboratory Registry") that identifies all poor performance laboratories. As CAP is not deemed to accredit in areas of genetics, it does not make the results of its assessments of genetic test performance public. **The Task Force recommends that CAP/ACMG periodically publish, and make available to the public, a list of laboratories performing genetic tests satisfactorily under its voluntary program.** Other PT programs should also publish the names of laboratories performing satisfactorily if they do not already do so. Directories of laboratories providing genetic tests should also publish information on listed laboratories' satisfactory participation in PT and other quality control programs specific to genetic tests. **Managed care organizations and other third-party payers should limit reimbursement for genetic tests to the laboratories on published lists of those satisfactorily performing genetic tests.**

A Central Repository of Cell Lines and DNA

Making cell lines or DNA containing disease-related mutations available to many laboratories would be useful in the validation of new tests, calibration, standardization, and quality control. To accomplish this, **appropriate specimens from patients, carriers, and controls should be available through a centralized repository in order to facilitate their availability to aid in analytical validation, improving quality, and other needs.**

<u>The Importance of the Pre- and Post-analytic Phases of Testing</u>

Educational and promotional material made available by laboratories is often used by providers and consumers who are considering testing. The completeness and accuracy of this material is, therefore, extremely important. Obtaining informed consent helps ensure that the person voluntarily agrees to testing and has some understanding of the reasons for testing. **The Task Force is of the opinion that laboratories should obtain documentation of informed consent when appropriate and should not perform an analysis if documentation is lacking.**

Increasingly, genetic tests will be requested by providers without much or any training in genetics. **Genetic test results must be written by the laboratory in a form that is understandable to the non-geneticist health care provider.**

<u>Local Review.</u> **The Task Force strongly suggests that any organization in which tests are developed conduct a structured review of the analytical and clinical validity and utility of new genetic tests before marketing them or otherwise making them available for clinical use. This structured review should be conducted by those not actually involved in developing the** CDC should consider how the pre- and post-analytic phases of predictive genetic testing can be given greater weight in CLIA standards and regulations.

<u>Direct Marketing of Genetic Tests to the Public</u>

Many clinical laboratories advertise the availability of tests directly to the public. **Great care must be taken that information on genetic tests presented directly to the public is accurate and includes risks and limitations, as well as benefits. Consumers should discuss testing options with a health care provider competent in genetics prior to having specimens collected for analysis. The Task Force discourages advertising or marketing of predictive genetic tests to the public.**

<u>International Harmonization</u>

The Task Force recommends that efforts should be made to harmonize international laboratory standards to ensure the highest possible laboratory quality for genetic tests.

IMPROVING PROVIDERS' UNDERSTANDINGS OF GENETIC TESTING

The rate of increase of health care professionals trained and board-certified in medical genetics or genetic counseling has not kept pace with the rate of increase of genetic discovery and of potential demand for genetic tests. Other health care professionals will have to play a role or new models of testing will have to be devised if the demands are to be met.

<u>A Role for Non-genetic Health Care Professionals</u>

With adequate knowledge of test validity, disease and mutation frequencies in the ethnic groups to whom they provide care, primary care providers and other non-genetic specialists can and should be the ones to offer predictive genetic tests to at-risk individuals. The role of non-genetic providers in interpreting test results is complex. The interpretation of positive results will often depend on further elicitation of risks, including family history. The options available to reduce risks must also be known. Often the results will be of importance to other relatives. A test's sensitivity and predictive value may also vary by ethnic group. Providers must be aware of these and other considerations in interpreting test results and be capable of communicating risk information and its implications to those who are tested or their parents or guardians. Consultation with geneticists and/or genetic counselors may be appropriate.

Policies for Improving the Abilities of Non-genetic Health Care Professionals
Greater Public Knowledge of Genetics. **A knowledge base on genetics and genetic testing should be developed for the general public.** Without a sound knowledge base, informed decisions are impossible and claims of autonomy and informed consent suspect. People who are more knowledgeable will grasp more readily the issues raised by providers when they offer tests. This could diminish the time needed for education and counseling without reducing consideration of the implications of testing. **New models of providing education and counseling to patients and other consumers are needed.**

Undergraduate and Graduate Medical Education. **The Task Force encourages the development of genetics curricula in medical school and residency training to enable all physicians to recognize inherited risk factors in patients and families and appreciate issues in genetic testing and the use of genetic services.** Those responsible for education and training have begun to recognize that most medical care is provided in ambulatory settings and that the delivery of care in those areas presents challenges for education. Genetic testing is a prime example. Moreover, teaching about genetic tests, including such issues as analytic and clinical validity, introduces students and residents to general problems of reliability and test sensitivity and specificity, which are important for a much wider range of clinical laboratory tests.

Licensure and Certification. **The likelihood that genetics will be covered in curricula will improve if relevant genetics questions are included in general licensure and specialty board certification examinations, and if correctly answering a proportion of the genetics questions is needed to attain a passing score.**

Continuing Medical Education. The full beneficial effects of improving medical school and residency curricula in genetics will not be felt for many years. Consequently, improving the ability of providers currently in practice to offer and interpret genetic tests correctly is of paramount importance. **In addition to the basic curricula already considered, the Task Force recommends that each specialty involved with the care of patients with disorders with genetic components should design its own curriculum for continuing education in genetics.**

Administrators and other nonphysician personnel who triage patients and/or make coverage or reimbursement decisions, such as those in managed care organizations, should also have knowledge of the benefits and risks of genetic testing.

The Task Force endorses the recent establishment of a National Coalition for Health Professional Education in Genetics (NCHPEG) by the American Medical Association, the American Nurses Association, and the National Human Genome Research Institute. In order to avoid duplication, the Coalition should serve as a registry and clearinghouse for, and disseminator of, information about various curricula and educational programs, grants, and training pilot programs in genetics education. It should encourage professional societies to track the effectiveness of their respective educational programs.

A major problem in all educational endeavors is finding the "teachable moment," the time at which people, including health care providers, are receptive to new information and are most likely to retain it. These moments arise when providers are asked questions about genetic tests or when charts are flagged because the patient fulfills criteria for being offered a genetic test. To make information available at the teachable moments, a 1-800 hotline that providers can call to learn more about specific genetic tests should be encouraged by NCHPEG.

<u>Demonstrating Provider Competence</u>. **Hospitals and managed care organizations, on advice from the relevant medical specialty departments, should request evidence of competence before permitting providers to order predictive genetic tests defined as needing stringent scrutiny or to counsel about them. Periodic, systematic medical record review, with feedback to providers, should also be used to ensure appropriate use of genetic tests.** In order to succeed, this policy requires, first, deciding which tests need evidence of competence, second, defining competence for those tests, and third, making educational modules readily available to enable providers to gain competence.

Medical record audits assure managed care and other organizations that providers are satisfying standards of care. The feedback given to providers also serves as a valuable reenforcement to what has previously been learned. Audits of records for frequently-ordered medical tests should be considered.

<u>Other Models</u>

<u>Nursing</u>. Nurses have much to offer in helping people before, during, and after the genetic testing process. Because of their vast numbers and the wide range of health care activities they can perform, they can play an important role in providing care for those undergoing genetic testing. Nurses should be provided with additional education and training that can increase their effectiveness in providing education for people undergoing genetic testing.

<u>Community and Public Health</u>. Although population-wide screening can be integrated into personal health care, different models have been used. In many states, it is the responsibility of the hospital in which the baby is born to conduct newborn screening. As tests for more inherited conditions become available and the safety and effectiveness of treating them neonatally is established, newborn screening could expand markedly.

Community-centered screening presents another model. Tay-Sachs carrier screening was originally organized at the community level. Any effort to initiate community-based genetic screening must have the support and involvement of the community. Particularly when minority communities are involved, the program must be sensitive to issues of discrimination and provide sufficient resources for education and counseling.

Screening could be offered in health department clinics, mobile vans or other sites, but not all segments of the population are likely to utilize them. A greater chance of breaching confidentiality is possible at community and health department sites than in the privacy of the traditional provider-patient relationship. Traditionally, health departments have been most involved in clinical care when there were well-accepted interventions (such as immunizations or tuberculosis control) without which the health of the public would be jeopardized. It might be difficult for public health personnel to appreciate that someone who refuses genetic screening is not jeopardizing the health of the public.

Before these new models are investigated, additional training of the personnel involved is necessary. **Schools of nursing, public health, and social work need to strengthen their training programs in genetics.**

GENETIC TESTING FOR RARE INHERITED DISORDERS

Between 10 and 20 million Americans may suffer from one or more of the several thousand known rare diseases over their lifetimes. With the discovery of the role of inherited mutations in common diseases, such as breast and colon cancer and Alzheimer disease (albeit in a small proportion of affected people), **the development and maintenance of tests for rare genetic diseases must continue to be encouraged. A comprehensive system to collect data on rare diseases must be established.** Multiple sources will almost always be needed to validate tests for rare diseases. CDC and the NIH Office of Rare Diseases (ORD) should work closely to develop the appropriate data-gathering and monitoring systems to assess the validity of genetic tests for rare diseases.

Dissemination of Information About Rare Diseases

Unfortunately, the diagnosis of rare diseases is often delayed. One reason for the delay is inaccessibility of information. **Physicians who encounter patients with symptoms and signs of rare genetic diseases should have access to accurate information that will enable them to include such diseases in their differential diagnosis, to know where to turn for assistance in clinical and laboratory diagnosis, and to locate laboratories that test for rare diseases.**

Several private and public organizations, both professional and consumer-oriented, do provide information on rare diseases. The Task Force is concerned that there might be some unnecessary duplication of effort in compiling databases while, at the same time, some diseases or laboratories offering tests will not be included. **In order to avoid redundancy and to use the expertise of these organizations more efficiently, NIH should assign its Office of Rare Diseases (ORD) the task of coordinating these efforts and provide ORD with sufficient funds to fulfill the Task Force's recommendations on rare diseases. ORD should periodically report to the proposed Secretary's Advisory Committee on the status of these activities.** With CDC playing a greater role in genetics, it should be closely involved in activities in this area.

Ensuring Continuity and Quality of Tests for Rare Diseases

Because of the rarity of many diseases, only one or a few laboratories in the United States, or the world, accurately perform tests for some of them. **To maintain and expand its database, ORD should identify laboratories worldwide that perform tests for rare genetic diseases, the methodology employed, and whether the tests they provide are in the investigational stage, or are being used for clinical diagnosis and decision making.**

Some clinical diagnostic tests for rare diseases are performed in laboratories that are primarily engaged in research at no cost to the patient and with the primary purpose of furthering research. Such laboratories may cease performing these tests, on which clinical decisions are based, as they complete their investigations and move on to other areas of interest. **The NIH Office of Rare Diseases should have the lead responsibility in ensuring the continued availability of safe and** effective tests for rare diseases when it learns that a test will cease being offered. **Funds to enable it to accomplish this task should be available.**

Ensuring the Quality of Genetic Tests for Rare Diseases

In accordance with current law, the Task Force recommends that any laboratory performing any genetic test on which clinical diagnostic and/or management decisions are made should be certified under CLIA. Research laboratories that are not currently providing genetic test results to providers or patients but that plan to do so in the future must register under CLIA. Once a laboratory registers, it does not have to wait for a survey before performing clinical tests.

Research laboratories that provide physicians with results of genetic tests, which may be used for clinical decision making, must validate their tests and be subject to the same internal and external review as other clinical laboratories. Nevertheless, the proposed genetics subcommittee of CLIAC should consider developing regulatory language under the proposed genetics specialty that is less stringent, but does not sacrifice quality for laboratories that only occasionally and in small volume perform tests whose results are made available to health care providers or patients.

Directories of laboratories that perform tests for rare genetic diseases should indicate whether or not the laboratory is CLIA-certified and whether it has satisfied other quality assessment and proficiency assessments, such as those provided by CAP and ACMG. Directors of these laboratories are encouraged to participate in these programs or other programs of at least comparable quality that may be established.

Of great concern to the Task Force is whether certification under CLIA will ensure the quality of genetic tests, particularly those for rare genetic diseases. The creation of a subspecialty of genetics under CLIA will greatly improve the situation. Many tests for rare disorders are biochemical. The quality of performance of these tests would be ensured if they were included under a genetics specialty.

CHAPTER 1. INTRODUCTION

The remarkable advances in genetics in recent decades are the fruition of almost a century of basic research. Our ability to identify the underlying defects in single-gene (Mendelian) diseases, most of which are rare, has improved diagnosis in symptomatic individuals, and the prediction of risks of future disease in asymptomatic individuals. We have learned how to prevent a few of these

---

Treatments for single gene (Mendelian) diseases. The interventions involve conventional therapies: pharmaceuticals, as in Wilson disease, congenital adrenal hyperplasia, and sickle cell anemia; special diets, as in phenylketonuria (PKU) and hereditary fructose intolerance, or such ancient and usually harmful practices as blood-letting (phlebotomy), as in hereditary hemochromatosis.[1] Recently, recombinant DNA techniques have made it possible to treat patients with hemophilia with recombinant human factor VIII, eliminating the fatal complication of acquired immunodeficiency syndrome and to treat patients with growth hormone deficiency with recombinant human growth hormone, eliminating the fatal complication of Creutzfeldt-Jacob disease. In both of these conditions, the complications resulted from extraction of the missing protein from human tissues.

---

diseases by early intervention and how to treat a few others after symptoms appear. Gene therapy, in which a normal gene is introduced into cells of patients with defective genes, is being investigated in over 1,000 individuals, including some with Mendelian disorders such as cystic fibrosis and adenosine deaminase deficiency.[2]

We now know that a small percentage of people with common disorders have inherited rare, single mutations that make them much more susceptible to developing the disease. Occasionally, single mutations that markedly increase susceptibility to disease reach frequencies as high as 1% in some population groups;[3] usually the <u>combined</u> frequency of all such mutations is under 5% of all those who will develop the disease. More common genetic variants (polymorphisms) less markedly increase susceptibility.

Over the past half century, scientists have discovered the existence of DNA polymorphisms in which the most common form (allele) occurs in no more than 99% of the population. We are beginning to learn that some of these polymorphisms are associated with increased risks of common diseases, but usually not to the same degree as the rare variants. Conversely, some forms of polymorphisms convey resistance to disease. Before disease develops in people with either predisposing rare variants or polymorphisms, other genetic and environmental factors must be present.

The role of genes in common diseases.

     <u>Rare variants</u>. Rare inherited variants (alleles) of single genes confer susceptibility to common diseases, such as BRCA1 and BRCA2 alleles for breast cancer,[4] alleles of four different DNA repair gene loci for hereditary nonpolyposis colon cancer,[5] and alleles in the presenilin and amyloid precursor protein genes for Alzheimer disease.[6] These alleles account for only a small proportion of all people with these diseases, and not all people with these variants will ever get the disease. Some alleles may occur more frequently in some ethnic groups, e.g. two alleles in the BRCA1 gene, which predispose to breast cancer, each occur in approximately 1% of Ashkenazi Jews.[3]

     <u>Polymorphisms</u>. A somewhat larger proportion of the common diseases are associated with more frequently occurring genetic polymorphisms (which occur in 1% or more of the population) but these polymorphisms do not usually confer as high a risk of disease as the rare single-gene variants. The E4 polymorphic form of apolipoprotein E is associated with an increased risk of Alzheimer disease,[7] histocompatibility gene variant HLA-Dqβ with insulin-dependent diabetes,[8,9] Factor V Leiden and the V polymorphism of methylene tetrahydrofolate reductase with venous thromboembolism,[10,11] and angiotensinogen-converting enzyme with cardiomyopathy.[12] Scientists have also discovered that the particular form of certain polymorphic genes we inherit affect our ability to absorb, transport, and metabolize drugs,[13] and respond to infectious agents such as HIV.[14] Increasingly, physicians will test for the inherited drug-handling capabilities of patients and use the results to tailor therapies for a wide range of diseases.[15]

     Genetic discovery can benefit people in other ways than by discovering the inherited components. In the case of cancer, scientists have learned that acquired (somatic) mutations play a significant role.[16] By comparing the molecular genetic profiles of cells from diseased organs and tissues to the comparable normal cells, scientists are beginning to learn which gene functions have been altered and how they might affect the development of chronic conditions like osteoporosis and arthritis.[17] With this knowledge, interventions can be devised to avert or treat the triggering events or treat the disease effectively in its early stages.

     Despite this remarkable progress much remains unknown. The unknowns have a strong impact on genetic testing, particularly when it is used predictively in healthy or apparently healthy people.

- No effective interventions are yet available to improve the outcome of most inherited diseases. It has proven far more difficult to devise a means of preventing or treating most Mendelian genetic diseases than to diagnose or predict increased risk of them. A "therapeutic gap" exists.

2

- Negative (normal) test results might not rule out future occurrence of disease. In the case of single-gene disorders, some tests do not detect all of the mutations capable of causing disease. In the case of common disorders, the disease often occurs even when tests for inherited susceptibility mutations or predisposing polymorphisms are negative.

- Positive test results might not mean the disease will inevitably develop. This is particularly a problem for the common disorders. For those who get the disease, the age at which it occurs and its severity and response to treatment cannot always be predicted. These problems arise in some Mendelian disorders, as well as in the common disorders. For instance, the severity of the lung disease, the most life-threatening aspect of cystic fibrosis, cannot be predicted by the mutations a person with CF possesses.[22]

> **The therapeutic gap: we can diagnose or predict disease but we can't treat or prevent it.** Extrapolating from a recent report on the proportion of genetic diseases for which interventions improve the outcome,[18] of the 674 single-gene diseases for which the underlying genetic defect had been discovered and reported, in about 80 (as of July 1997 in Online Mendelian Inheritance in Man, http://www.ncbi.nlm.nih.gov/Omim) we could expect the prognosis to have been improved significantly. Partial improvement could be expected in about 360. For more common disorders, early interventions for some types of inherited colon cancer do improve outcomes,[19] but the effectiveness of interventions to prevent breast or ovarian cancer, or detect them earlier in those with inherited susceptibility mutations, is just beginning to be studied.[20,21] For many other disorders, no therapy is yet available.

It is primarily in the context of their unknown potential risks and benefits that the Task Force considers genetic testing.

Research and discovery in the first century of the next millennium will reduce the uncertainties, but the nature of human variation is such that it will never be possible to have genetic tests that are perfect predictors of disease. Even today, however, tests for the disorders for which these problems have not been solved can be of benefit.

- A negative test result in someone from a family in which affected relatives are known to have a disease-related mutation indicates a low risk of the disease. This can decrease anxiety and, for some diseases, reduce the frequency of periodic monitoring for early signs of the disease (e.g., mammography for breast cancer). A negative result can, depending on the disease, also enable a person to purchase health or life insurance at the standard rate.

- A positive test result enables a person to prepare for disease. Parents who learn from carrier screening that they are at risk of having an affected child can take steps to avoid the conception or birth of an affected child. People at risk of disease later in life can take steps to avoid passing the disease-causing allele on to their future children or can plan for the disease.

- Knowing that one is a carrier or has inherited a susceptibility to disease enables the person to inform relatives that they also might be at risk.

In the absence of treatment, some people will be deterred from testing.
- Some people would prefer not to know their individual risks.
- Some people would prefer not to know risks to their future children because under no circumstances would they attempt to avoid the conception or the birth of an affected child.
- Some people would prefer not to tell relatives of their own risk or the possible risk to their relatives.
- Knowing that one is likely to get a disease that might have a protracted course because no effective treatment is available might prevent some people from getting health insurance, or require them to pay a higher premium, or have the condition excluded from coverage. They might also be denied jobs because of their risk of future disease.
- People who have a greater chance of dying early might be denied life insurance or have to pay a higher premium.
- Some people will fear that their test results will be accessible to others whom they do not wish to have the information.

Nevertheless, problems will remain, especially as long as the means of preventing or treating genetic disease in those born with it are not fully at hand. The Task Force was created to make recommendations to ensure that genetic tests are safe and effective in view of the persistence of problems in the foreseeable future.

ORIGIN AND WORK OF THE TASK FORCE

In 1994, the National Institutes of Health (NIH)-Department of Energy (DOE) Working Group on Ethical, Legal, and Social Implications (ELSI) of Human Genome Research reviewed the report of the Institute of Medicine's Committee on Assessing Genetic Risks.[23] Among the concerns raised in that report were the imperfect predictability of tests, the quality of laboratories providing clinical genetic tests, the lack of proven interventions for many disorders (see chapter 3), and the limited ability of many health care providers to explain genetic tests accurately and nondirectively to patients (see chapter 4). To consider these problems further, the Working Group convened the Task Force on Genetic Testing. It asked the Task Force to review genetic testing in the United States and, when necessary, make recommendations to ensure the development of safe and effective genetic tests. The Task Force has defined safety and effectiveness to encompass not only the validity and utility of genetic tests, but their delivery in laboratories of assured quality, and their appropriate use by health care providers and consumers.

4

How the public in general should be educated in genetics and genetic testing is beyond the purview of the Task Force, although it is critically important. So too, are policy recommendations-- other than for improving genetic tests themselves--for reducing the harms that can result from some forms of genetic testing and can deter some people from being tested. Nevertheless, later in this chapter, the Task Force enunciates principles related to these harms.

The Working Group invited organizations with a stake in genetic testing to submit nominations from which it selected members of the Task Force. In addition, the Working Group invited five agencies in the Department of Health and Human Services (HHS) to send nonvoting liaison members to the Task Force. (Task Force members and their affiliations are listed at the front of this report.)

To determine the state of the art of genetic testing in the U.S., a survey of organizations likely to be engaged in genetic testing was undertaken for the Task Force early in 1995. Following completion of the survey, in-depth interviews were conducted at 29 of the 463 organizations that indicated they were developing or providing genetic tests. Informational materials for providers and patients that were distributed by respondents who were performing genetic tests were collected and analyzed. Appendix 3 of the final report is a summary of the survey and interview findings, and appendix 4 is a summary of the analysis of the informational materials. The Task Force also commissioned papers on some of the more frequent genetic screening programs in the U.S. These appear in appendices 5 and 6. With the help of liaison representatives of relevant agencies and others, Task Force staff prepared analyses of various Federal statutes and regulations, most importantly those dealing with clinical laboratories and medical devices. Through notices in various genetics journals, an announcement on its World Wide Web page, and requests to consumer organizations, the Task Force asked professionals and consumers to report their experiences with various aspects of genetic testing. A small number of genetic counselors, physicians, and affected patients or their relatives responded. Some of these responses appear as sidebars throughout this report.

In this report, all principles and recommendations of the Task Force appear in **bold-faced type.** Unfamiliar terminology can be found in the glossary.

The Task Force recognizes the tremendous potential of benefits from genetic testing. Its goal is to make recommendations that will assure the public that genetic tests will be safe and effective but will not stifle progress in this exciting field. It is particularly concerned about the continued availability of tests for rare inherited diseases.

The Task Force held seven meetings, all of which were open to the public. Halfway through its deliberations, the Task Force published Interim Principles,[24] made them available on its World Wide Web site (http://ww2.med.jhu.edu/tfgtelsi), invited public comments, and held a public hearing on them. Taking these comments into consideration, the Task Force turned to developing recommendations to implement its principles. These were published in the Federal Register and also made available on the Web site.[25] Once again, the public was given an opportunity to comment. A list of all organizations and persons commenting on the Interim Principles and Proposed Recommendations appears in appendix 1 of this report. The Task Force has taken these comments into consideration in preparing its final principles and recommendations.

DEFINITION OF GENETIC TESTS

The Task Force could not make recommendations on genetic tests without first defining them. After hearing considerable comment and much deliberation, the Task Force developed the following definition.

Genetic test--The analysis of human DNA, RNA, chromosomes, proteins, and certain metabolites in order to detect inherited disease-related genotypes, mutations, phenotypes, or karyotypes for clinical purposes. Such purposes include predicting risk of disease, identifying carriers, and establishing prenatal and clinical diagnosis or prognosis. Prenatal, newborn and carrier screening, as well as testing in high risk families, are included. Tests for metabolites are covered only when they are undertaken with high probability that an excess or deficiency of the metabolite indicates the presence of inherited mutations in single genes. Tests conducted purely for research[a] are excluded from the definition, as are tests for somatic (as opposed to inherited) mutations, and testing for forensic purposes.

The Task Force is primarily concerned about predictive uses of genetic tests performed in healthy or apparently healthy people. Predictive test results do not necessarily mean that the disease will inevitably occur or remain absent; they replace the individual's prior risks based on population data or family history with risks based on genotype. The Task Force divides predictive tests into presymptomatic tests, which are performed to detect highly "penetrant" conditions, and predispositional tests, which are performed for incompletely penetrant conditions. The Task Force cannot limit its definition to predictive tests because some tests intended for diagnostic use can also be used predictively. The Task Force also decided that it cannot limit genetic tests only to those for which the analyte is DNA. Clinical laboratories will continue to use protein and enzyme and metabolite analyses for the purposes listed in the definition, including prediction.

Some, but not all, predictive genetic testing falls under the rubric "genetic screening." The Task Force follows the definition used in a National Research Council report: "Genetic screening may be defined as a search in a population for persons possessing certain genotypes that (1) are already associated with disease or predispose to disease, (2) may lead to disease in their descendants, or (3) produce other variations not known to be associated with disease." [26 (p. 9)] Under this definition, testing an asymptomatic person in a family with several relatives affected with disease does not constitute screening but predictive genetic testing.

The Task Force rejected the suggestion from the College of American Pathologists (CAP) that, "The definition of genetic tests should focus on germ line mutations that require genetic counseling with respect to the development of diseases."[b] Neither the Task Force nor any other body has stated which tests require genetic counseling. The Task Force did acknowledge the concerns of CAP and The American Society of Clinical Pathologists that too many tests in standard use would be covered by limiting its definition to tests for metabolites only when they are "undertaken with high

---

[a]Tests conducted purely for research are those in which test results are not given to patients or their providers under any circumstances.

[b]R.C. Zastrow, President, College of American Pathologists, Communication to the Task Force, May 30, 1996.

6

probability that an excess or deficiency of the metabolite indicates the presence of inherited mutations in single genes". Under the definition, cholesterol screening in the general population would not be covered, but cholesterol testing in a family with a documented low density lipoprotein receptor defect would be covered. Newborn screening tests for metabolites whose excess or deficiency require followup to rule out a heritable disorder would be covered.

It is not the intention of the Task Force that all of its recommendations be applied to all tests that meet its definition. A system is needed to classify genetic tests according to the scrutiny they need. Later in this chapter, the Task Force suggests how such a system can be developed.

REVIEW OF GENETIC TESTING

Over 500 commercial, university, and health department laboratories provide tests for inherited and chromosomal disorders, and genetic predispositions in the United States. Virtually every newborn is screened for phenylketonuria and congenital hypothyroidism and many are screened for sickle cell disorders.[27] Screening for carriers of Tay-Sachs and sickle cell is performed among populations at risk. Based on the recommendations of a recent consensus panel,[28] cystic fibrosis carrier screening might increase. Approximately 2.5 million pregnant women are screened each year to see if their fetuses are at high risk of neural tube defects or Down syndrome.[29] Of 467 organizations who responded fully to the survey conducted for the Task Force, 56.7% indicated that they were testing for at least one of 44 inherited conditions that were listed in the questionnaire (see appendix 3). A few commercial and university laboratories were offering tests for inherited susceptibility mutations to breast and colon cancer. Of 197 health maintenance organizations who responded to a recent survey, 45% said they were covering predictive tests for breast cancer and 42% were covering for colon cancer for some of their subscribers.[30]

For the most part, genetic testing in the United States has developed successfully, providing options for avoiding, preventing, and treating inherited disorders. However, there are some problems, which are spelled out in greater detail later in this report and in the appendices.

- Sometimes, genetic tests are introduced before they have been demonstrated to be safe, effective, and useful (see chapter 2 and appendices 5 and 6).
- There is no assurance that every laboratory performing genetic tests for clinical purposes meets high standards (see chapter 3).
- Often, the informational materials distributed by academic and commercial genetic testing laboratories do not provide sufficient information to fill in the gaps in providers' and patients' understanding of genetic tests (see appendix 4).

THE NEED FOR RECOMMENDATIONS

In the past few years, scientific and professional societies, as well as consumer groups, have felt impelled to publicly express concern when predictive tests were introduced with insufficient evidence of safety and effectiveness. These included prenatal screening with alpha-fetoprotein and other markers,[31,32] carrier screening for cystic fibrosis,[33,34] testing for susceptibility to cancer[35,36] and breast cancer in particular,[37,38] and Alzheimer disease.[39,40] These statements often expressed a reaction to the imminence or appearance of a test and undoubtedly reduced inappropriate use of tests. The publication of each statement depended on mobilizing individuals with interest and expertise and then getting ratification by the sponsoring organization, tasks not easily accomplished in a short period without extraordinary effort. This becomes an impossible task as the number of tests expands but the problems persist.

Although professional societies must play a major role in solving problems of genetic testing, they are only one of several stakeholders, some of whose interests conflict with others'. The Task Force believes that all stakeholders must be involved. As this report demonstrates, they often will succeed in resolving disagreements and reaching consensus.

Except for neonatal and prenatal screening and diagnosis, the volume of testing has not been great and much of the testing has been performed in genetic centers or in consultation with highly-trained geneticists and genetic counselors. In the next few years, the use of genetic testing is likely to expand rapidly while the number of genetic specialists remains essentially unchanged. A greater

---

Directiveness in counseling. "After being asked repeatedly if we would have had our children if we had known they had NF (Neurofibromatosis 2), I finally asked...those who worked with us to please stop asking. My oldest child had reached the age when she understood the implications of the question, and we had heard it and answered it enough times to last us several life-times. Our experiences with several doctors has been that they are appalled that we could bring into this world children who were at risk of having NF. Other doctors have talked down to us as if we must certainly have just been stupid to even consider having children...It is our firm belief that God makes the decisions of whether or not to bless people with children. We consider all three of our children to be blessings, even the two with NF. Our concerns about genetic research (include)...that women will be pressured to have abortions if they have genetically defective babies. Think of the famous scientists, presidents and others who might not have been born if their genetic defects were known before their births."--Woman whose husband and two of three children have NF.

---

burden for making genetic testing decisions will fall on providers who have little formal training or experience in genetics and are less equipped to deal with the complex and special problems raised by some predictive genetic tests. Consulted primarily by people who are sick, and who expect doctors to tell them what to do to get better, many physicians adopt a directive stance when asked how they would deal with genetic tests and results that have reproductive implications.

Until the 1980s most genetic and cytogenetic testing was performed in the laboratories of non-profit organizations, most of them in academic medical centers. These labs were often directed by the same professionals who cared for patients. In the last decade, genetic testing has been commercialized. As a result, providers who were close to patients and families at risk of illness might not have as much influence on testing policy as they once did.

8

Although formal comparisons have not been made, there is little evidence that the problems encountered in the development and delivery of genetic testing technologies have been more frequent or severe than for other medical technologies. Some problems encountered in other specialties have not been trivial. Amendments to the Food, Drug and Cosmetic Act, and to the Clinical Laboratory Improvement Act were passed by Congress because of problems in the clinical use of some new medical technologies.[41-45] In 1996, recognizing the challenge posed by genetic tests, two Congressional committees held hearings related to the validity and quality of genetic tests.[46,47]

Commercial interest in genetic testing. In the survey conducted for the Task Force, 147 biotechnology companies reported that they were engaged in genetic testing activities, including 58 who were developing or marketing genetic tests and an additional 89 who were performing research or developing ancillary products. Biotechnology companies were significantly more likely than nonprofit university laboratories to be developing or offering tests for common disorders (see appendix 3).

The ELSI component of the Human Genome Project was founded on the concept that the new technologies of gene identification will engender problems that can be minimized if anticipated and dealt with promptly. The recommendations of the Task Force are very much in this vein. In this report, the Task Force does not recommend policies for specific tests but suggests a framework for ensuring that new tests meet criteria for safety and effectiveness before they are unconditionally released, thereby reducing the likelihood of premature clinical use.

The focus of the Task Force on potential problems in no way is intended to detract from the benefits of genetic testing. Its overriding goal is to recommend policies that will reduce the likelihood of damaging effects so testing's benefits can be fully realized undiluted by harm.

SCOPE OF THE REPORT

The Task Force has tried to stay within the limits of its charge and to use past and current genetic testing as its guide. In the remainder of this chapter we consider the need for a central advisory body on genetic testing, and enunciate overarching principles on problems that are not integral to genetic testing per se but impinge on, or that may arise as a consequence of, genetic testing. The next chapter considers criteria for the development of new genetic tests. It presents policies to ensure that sufficient evidence of the safety and effectiveness of new genetic tests is collected and is reviewed before tests are unconditionally made available for clinical use. In chapter 3, we consider how the quality of the laboratories that provide genetic testing to health care providers in clinical practice can be ensured. Because new tests are often developed in clinical laboratories, the chapter begins with a consideration of laboratories' responsibilities in developing new tests. In chapter 4, the expanding role of non-genetic health care providers in genetic testing is considered, followed by discussion of some of the obstacles to their providing testing appropriately. The chapter describes policies to ensure that providers who use genetic testing have an adequate understanding of the indications for genetic tests and their limitations. Chapter 5 raises several concerns about rare genetic diseases, which constitute the largest number of genetic diseases. Collectively rare diseases represent the most frequent indication for genetic testing. Policies for ensuring that providers include rare diseases when they consider the causes of some of their patients' problems and that they know how and where to obtain information about rare diseases, including where to obtain diagnostic and predictive clinical laboratory tests, are considered. The chapter concludes with recommendations for ensuring the continuity and quality of clinical laboratory tests, for rare diseases. Chapter 6 presents those recommendations the Task Force wishes to highlight.

This report does not contain a separate chapter on genetic testing under public health auspices. The Task Force spent considerable time discussing this issue and concluded that its recommendations for genetic tests in clinical practice also apply to tests included in health department screening programs. Some members of the Task Force and several who submitted comments questioned the need for informed consent in public health programs that are undertaken only when the benefits to the individual markedly outweigh the risks. Task Force principles on this issue are presented later in this chapter. A public health role is discussed briefly in chapter 4.

NEED FOR AN ADVISORY COMMITTEE ON GENETIC TESTING

Policies related to genetic testing involve several different Federal agencies, as well as the private sector. Such policies can best be formulated and implemented by having input from many different sources in order to achieve the single goal: the availability of safe and effective genetic tests.

The Task Force calls on the Secretary of Health and Human Services to establish an advisory committee on genetic testing in the Office of the Secretary. Members of the committee should represent the stakeholders in genetic testing, including professional societies (general medicine, genetics, pathology, genetic counseling), the biotechnology industry, consumers, and insurers, as well as other interested parties. The various HHS agencies with activities related to the development and delivery of genetic tests should send nonvoting representatives to the advisory committee, which can also coordinate the relevant activities of these agencies and private organizations. The Task Force leaves it to the Secretary to determine the relationship of this advisory committee to others that may be created in the broader area of genetics and public policy, of which genetic testing is only one part.

The committee would advise the Secretary on implementation of recommendations made by the Task Force in this report to ensure that (a) the introduction of new genetic tests into clinical use is based on evidence of their analytical and clinical validity, and utility to those tested; (b) all stages of the genetic testing process in clinical laboratories meet quality standards; (c) health providers who offer and order genetic tests have sufficient competence in genetics and genetic testing to protect the well-being of their patients; and (d) there be continued and expanded availability of tests for rare genetic diseases.

The Task Force recognizes the widely inclusive nature of genetic tests. It is therefore essential that the advisory committee recommend policies for the Secretary's consideration by which agencies and organizations implementing recommendations can determine those genetic tests that need stringent scrutiny. Stringent scrutiny is indicated when a test has the ability

---

Functions of the proposed Secretary's Advisory Committee on Genetic Testing.
- Establish criteria for determining which tests need stringent scrutiny (see this chapter).
- Advise the Office for the Protection of Human Subjects from Research Risks (OPRR) and institutional review boards (IRBs) on criteria for reviewing protocols for genetic test development (giving priority to tests requiring stringent scrutiny) (see chapter 2, p. 31).
- Advise OPRR on streamlining the requirements for IRB review of multicenter collaborative protocols for genetic test development (see chapter 2, p. 33).
- Consider how national review of new genetic tests (for which data have been collected under IRB-approved protocols), especially those requiring stringent scrutiny, can be accomplished. Suggest criteria for review (see chapter 2, p. 38).
- Enhance communication and consistency in genetic testing activities across government agencies and private organizations (see this chapter).
- Work with FDA to harmonize definitions of stringent scrutiny, particularly as they relate to the classification of genetic testing devices (see chapter 2).
- Work with the Genetics Subcommittee of the Clinical Laboratory Improvement Advisory Committee to ensure quality of clinical laboratories performing genetic tests (see chapter 3, p. 41).
- Work with the National Coalition for Health Professional Education in Genetics to develop guidelines for assessing competence of non-genetic providers of genetic services (see chapter 4, p. 70).
- Work with the National Institutes of Health (NIH) Office of Rare Diseases to improve availability of information on rare genetic diseases, including clinical laboratory testing, for health care providers and consumers (see chapter 5, p. 81).

---

to predict future inherited disease in healthy or apparently healthy people, is likely to be used for that purpose, and when no confirmatory test is available. The advisory committee or its designate should define additional indications.

In order to carry out its functions, the advisory committee should have its own staff and budget.

The Task Force further recommends that the Secretary review the accomplishments of the advisory committee on genetic testing after 2 full years of operation and determine whether it should continue to operate.

NOTE: Hereafter, the advisory committee on genetic testing is referred to as the proposed Secretary's Advisory Committee.

OVERARCHING PRINCIPLES

In making recommendations on safety and effectiveness, the Task Force concentrated on test validity and utility, laboratory quality, and provider competence. It recognizes, however, that other issues impinge on testing, and problems can arise from testing. Regarding these issues, the Task Force endorses the following principles.

Informed Consent

The Task Force strongly advocates written informed consent, especially for certain uses of genetic tests, including clinical validation studies and predictive testing. The failure of the Task Force to comment on informed consent for other uses does not imply that it should not be obtained.

Test Development. **Informed consent for any validation study must be obtained whenever the specimen can be linked to the subject from which it came.** As long as identifiers are retained in either coded or uncoded form, the possibility exists to contact subjects even if the intent of the original protocol was not to do so. As part of the disclosure for consent, individuals must be informed of possible future uses of the specimen, whether identifiers will be retained and, if so, whether the individual will be recontacted.

Testing in Clinical Practice. **(1) It is unacceptable to coerce or intimidate individuals or families regarding their decision about predictive genetic testing. Respect for personal autonomy is paramount. People being offered testing must understand that testing is voluntary. Their informed consent should be obtained. Whatever decision they make, their care should not be jeopardized.** Information on risks and benefits must be presented fully and objectively. A non-directive approach is of the utmost importance when reproductive decisions are a consequence of testing or when the safety and effectiveness of interventions following a positive test result have not been established. Obtaining written informed consent helps to ensure that the person voluntarily agrees to testing.

(2) Prior to the initiation of predictive testing in clinical practice, health care providers must describe the features of the genetic test, including potential consequences, to potential test recipients. Individuals considering genetic testing must be told the purposes of the test, the chance it will give a correct prediction, the implications of test results, the options, and the benefits and risks of the process. The responsibility for providing information to the individual lies with the referring provider, not with the laboratory performing the test.

Newborn Screening. **(1) If informed consent is waived for a newborn screening test, the analytical and clinical validity and clinical utility of the test must be established, and parents must be provided with sufficient information to understand the reasons for screening.** By clinical utility, the Task Force means that interventions to improve the outcome of the infant identified by screening have been proven to be safe and effective. Using newborn screening to identify couples who are at risk of having a future child with sickle cell anemia or other disorder because their screened infant is found to be a carrier (heterozygote) is not of primary benefit to the infant screened. Using newborn screening to identify parents at risk should only be done after this intention is communicated to parents (prior to screening) and their written consent is obtained. The Task Force recognizes that newborn screening programs have succeeded in significantly reducing the burden of a number of inherited disorders by timely diagnosis and institution of preventive therapies.

Sometimes, however, newborn screening is undertaken before tests are validated and interventions are established to prevent or reduce clinical problems (see appendix 5). A recent consensus development conference on cystic fibrosis concluded that the evidence to warrant routine screening of newborns for cystic fibrosis was insufficient.[28]

(2) For those disorders for which newborn screening is available but the tests have not been validated or shown to have clinical utility, written parental consent is required prior to testing. The Task Force also recognizes that specimens collected for newborn screening become an important resource for developing new tests. When the infant's name or other identifying information is retained on these specimens, the Task Force believes that parental informed consent is needed.

Prenatal and Carrier Testing

Respect for an individual's/couples' beliefs and values concerning tests undertaken for assisting reproductive decisions is of paramount importance and can best be maintained by a nondirective stance. One way of ensuring that a non-directive stance is taken and that parents' decisions are autonomous, is through requiring informed consent.

Testing of Children

Genetic testing of children for adult onset diseases should not be undertaken unless direct medical benefit will accrue to the child and this benefit would be lost by waiting until the child has reached adulthood. The Task Force agrees with the American Society of Human Genetics and the American College of Medical Genetics that "Timely medical benefit to the child should be the primary justification for genetic testing in children and adolescents."[48] Although sympathetic to the considerable difficulties parents may have in living with uncertainty about the health status of the child, the Task Force does not feel that these warrant foreclosing the child's right to make an independent decision in regard to testing when the child reaches adulthood. We are aware, however, that there are situations (e.g., testing for inherited mutations in the adenomatous polyposis coli gene) in which the benefit of avoiding medical surveillance (if the test result is negative) is sufficient to warrant testing even though no treatment will usually be undertaken until a later age (if the test result is positive). In addition, the Task Force realizes that legal adulthood is a somewhat arbitrary concept. For example, in families with a considerable burden of disease and in which several adults are undergoing genetic testing, older teenagers might request testing for themselves in order to reduce uncertainty and anxiety. It is unfortunate that almost no research evidence currently exists on the risks and benefits of genetic testing to teenagers and younger children. We believe that such psychosocial research must be pursued as vigorously as research on issues of analytical and clinical validity or utility of tests. However, unless and until such time as contradictory research findings emerge, testing of minors for presumed psychological benefits should be avoided.

Confidentiality

Protecting the confidentiality of information is essential for all uses of genetic tests.

(1) Results should be released only to those individuals for whom the test recipient has given consent for information release. Means of transmitting information should be chosen to minimize the likelihood that results will become available to unauthorized persons or organizations. Under no circumstances should results with identifiers be provided to any

outside parties, including employers, insurers, or government agencies, without the test recipient's written consent. Consent given for minors should expire when the minor reaches adulthood.

Unless potential test recipients can be assured that the results will not be given to individuals or organizations they have not specifically named, some will refuse testing for fear of losing insurance, employment, or for other reasons. Aggregate results, stripped of identifiers, can be reported to government agencies for statistical and planning purposes.

(2) Health care providers have an obligation to the person being tested not to inform other family members without the permission of the person tested, except in extreme circumstances.

The Task Force agrees with recommendations of The President's Commission for the Study of Ethical Problems in Medicine and Biomedical and Behavioral Research[49] and the Institute of Medicine[23] that disclosure by providers to other family members is appropriate only when the person tested refuses to communicate information despite reasonable attempts to persuade him or her to do so, and when failure to give that information has a high probability of resulting in imminent, serious, and irreversible harm to the relative, and when communication of the information will enable the relative to avert the harm. When test results have serious implications for relatives, it is incumbent upon providers to explain to people who are tested the reasons why they should communicate the information to their relatives and to counsel them on how they should convey the information so the communication itself does not result in undue harm. Great care must be taken to avoid inadvertent release of information.

> **Confidentiality in testing relatives.** "I cannot tell you how many laboratories produce very nicely worded reports with the entire pedigree present so the counselor can interpret the results clearly. The problem is that the couple in front of you might also discover Aunt Minnie's status too...(L)abs should produce individual reports, one per person rather than one per family."--Genetic counselor

Recently, a subcommittee of the American Society of Human Genetics[50] endorsed these same principles for disclosure to relatives, but suggested that "the health care professional should be obliged to inform the patient of the implications of his/her genetic test results and potential risks to family members. *Prior to genetic testing* and again upon refusal to communicate results, this *duty to inform* the patient of familial implications is *paramount*. (emphasis added)." The Task Force is of the opinion that, as part of this duty, providers must make clear that they will not communicate results to relatives, except in extreme circumstances, which the provider should define. If left with the impression that the provider will inform relatives when the person considering testing does not want them informed, some people will decline testing. This would have the effect not only of denying information to the relative but to the person offered testing as well. Providers should be explicit in describing the extreme situations in which they would inform other relatives.

> **People may not always communicate appropriately to their relatives.** The asymptomatic father of an 18-year-old daughter, from whom he was estranged, had a positive test result for a very rare fatal disorder, for which he was at 50% risk. In giving him the positive result, his specialist advised him to arrange testing for his daughter and gave him request forms. The father contacted the daughter who had not been aware of the family history and she had the test performed in the same laboratory that tested the father. Despite the fact she was an adult, her positive result was not reported to her but given to her father who then told her. The daughter was referred to a genetics center for counseling after she told her primary care doctor, "...my whole future has fallen apart. I feel I can make no plans about employment, marriage or family. I was not warned about how I might react."--Abridged from a report from a geneticist who saw the young woman.

Harm can also result when relatives communicate genetic information. Strategies to assist individuals in communicating information to relatives should be developed.

Discrimination

No individual should be subjected to unfair discrimination by a third party on the basis of having had a genetic test or receiving an abnormal genetic test result. Third parties include insurers, employers, and educational and other institutions that routinely inquire about the health of applicants for services or positions. Discrimination can take the form of denial or of additional charges for various types of insurance, employment jeopardy in hiring and firing, or requirements to undergo unwanted genetic testing. Protection from unfair discrimination has been the subject of legislation at both the State and Federal levels.[51] The problem has not been completely solved.[52,53]

Consumer Involvement in Policy Making

Although other stakeholders are concerned about protecting consumers, they cannot always provide the perspective brought by consumers themselves, the end users of genetic testing. Clearly, there are technical issues that cannot be decided primarily by consumers, but consumers must be involved in decision making on matters of policy in test development and in clinical use that directly affects their well-being. **Consumers should be involved in policy (but not necessarily in technical) decisions regarding the adoption, introduction, and use of new, predictive genetic tests.**

Issues Not Covered

There are aspects of genetic testing with which we have not dealt. Several respondents asked the Task Force to comment on genetic testing for non-medical conditions, such as homosexuality or other behavioral traits, or for gene enhancement. Although the Task Force has drawn upon examples of past and current testing, it has not made pronouncements about specific types of testing. As already stated, its intent is to develop generic policies that cover predictive testing for a wide range of medical conditions.

The Task Force recognizes that patenting and licensing can have a profound effect on the costs of medical tests. The payment of license fees is likely to be passed on to third-party payers, or to consumers if they do not have or wish to use their health insurance. This issue has been highlighted recently by lawsuits by a patent holder to force laboratories performing prenatal screening for Down syndrome to pay royalties.[54] The issue of patenting and licensing needs further exploration but is beyond the scope of the Task Force.

The Task Force has not dwelled in depth on the use of stored tissues for genetic research, including the development of genetic tests. Recommendations on this issue have been made by others[55-58] and are still being actively discussed and modified.

Undoubtedly, others would have liked us to comment on additional issues. We reiterate that our main concern is the safety and effectiveness of genetic tests in both the developmental phase and the clinical-use phase. We turn now to these major topics.

REFERENCES

1. Scriver CR, Beaudet AL, Sly WS, Valle D, editors: *The Metabolic and Molecular Bases of Inherited Disease. Seventh Edition.* New York, McGraw-Hill, Inc. 1995.

2. Friedmann T: Overcoming the obstacles to gene therapy. *Scientific American* 1997;276:96-101.

3. Struewing JP, Hartge P, Wacholder S, et al: The risk of cancer associated with specific mutations of BRCA1 and BRCA2 among Ashkenazi Jews. *New England Journal of Medicine* 1997;336:1401-1408.

4. Szabo CI, King M: Invited editorial: Population genetics of BRCA1 and BRCA2. *American Journal of Human Genetics* 1997;60:1013-1020.

5. Kinzler KW, Vogelstein B: Lessons from hereditary colorectal cancer. *Cell* 1996;87:159-170.

6. Morrison-Bogorad M, Phelps C, Buckholtz N: Alzheimer disease research comes of age. The pace accelerates. *JAMA* 1997;277:837-840.

7. Seshadri S, Drachman DA, Lippa CF: Apolipoprotein E e4 allele and the lifetime risk of Alzheimer's disease. What physicians know, and what they should know. *Archives of Neurology* 1995;52:1074-1079.

8. Tisch R, McDevitt H: Insulin-dependent diabetes mellitus. *Cell* 1996;85:291-297.

9. Vyse TJ, Todd JA: Genetic analysis of autoimmune diseases. *Cell* 1996;85:311-318.

10. Ridker PM, Miletich JP, Hennekens CH, Buring JE: Ethnic distribution of Factor V Leiden in 4047 men and women. Implications for venous thromboembolism screening. *JAMA* 1997;277:1305-1307.

11. Frosst P, Blom HJ, Milos R, et al: A candidate genetic risk factor for vascular disease: A common mutation in methylenetetrahydrofolate reductase. *Nature Genetics* 1995;10:111-113.

12. Reynolds MV, Bristow MR, Bush EW, et al: Angiotensin-converting enzyme DD genotype in patients with ischaemic or idiopathic dilated cardiomyopathy. *Lancet* 1993;342:1073-1075.

13. Nebert DW: Polymorphisms in drug-metabolizing enzymes: What is their clinical relevance and why do they exist? *American Journal of Human Genetics* 1997;60:265-271.

14. Smith MW, Dean M, Carrington M, et al: Contrasting genetic influence of CCR2 and CCR5 variants on HIV-1 infection and disease progression. *Science* 1997;277:959-968.

15. Bell J: The new genetics of clinical practice. *BMJ* 1997;(In Press).

16. Vogelstein B, Kinzler KW: The multistep nature of cancer. *Trends in Genetics* 1993;9:138-141.

17. Haseltine WA: Discovering genes for new medicine. *Scientific American* 1997;276:92-97.

18. Treacy E, Childs B, Scriver CR: Response to treatment in hereditary metabolic disease: 1993 survey and 10-year comparison. *American Journal of Human Genetics* 1995;56:359-367.

19. Burke W, Petersen G, Lynch P, et al: Recommendations for follow-up care of individuals with an inherited predisposition to cancer. I. Hereditary nonpolyposis colon cancer. *JAMA* 1997;277:915-919.

20. Schrag D, Kuntz KM, Garber JE, Weeks JC: Decision analysis -- effects of prophylactic mastectomy and oophorectomy on life expectancy among women with BRCA1 or BRCA2 mutations. *New England Journal of Medicine* 1997;336:1465-1471.

21. Burke W, Daly M, Garber J, et al: Recommendations for follow-up care of individuals with an inherited predisposition to cancer. II. BRCA1 and BRCA2. *JAMA* 1997;277:997-1003.

22. Cystic Fibrosis Genotype-Phenotype Consortium: Correlation between genotype and phenotype in patients with cystic fibrosis. *New England Journal of Medicine* 1993;329:1308-1313.

23. Andrews L, Fullarton JE, Holtzman NA, Motulsky AG, eds. *Assessing genetic risks: Implications for health and social policy.* Washington DC, National Academy Press; 1994.

24. Task Force on Genetic Testing: Interim principles. *Available at www.med.jhu.edu/tfgtelsi* 1996.

25. National Institutes of Health: Proposed recommendations of the Task Force on Genetic Testing; Notice of meeting and request for comment. *Federal Register* 1997;62:4539-4547.

26. Committee for the Study of Inborn Errors of Metabolism: *Genetic screening: Programs, principles, and research.* Washington DC, National Academy of Sciences; 1975.

27. Hiller EH, Landenburger G, Natowicz MR: Public participation in medical policy making and the status of consumer autonomy: The example of newborn screening programs in the United States. *American Journal of Public Health* 1997;87(8):1280-1288.

28. Howell RR, Borecki I, Davidson ME, et al: National Institutes of Health Consensus Development Conference Statement: Genetic testing for cystic fibrosis. 1997;in press.

29. Palomaki GE, Knight GJ, McCarthy JE, Haddow JE, Donhowe JM: Maternal serum screening for Down syndrome in the United States: A 1995 survey. *American Journal of Obstetrics and Gynecology* 1997;176:1046-1051.

30. Myers MF, Doksum T, Holtzman NA: Coverage and provision of genetic services: Surveys of health maintenance organizations (HMOs) and academic genetic units (AGUs). *American Journal of Human Genetics* 1997;61(4, Supplement):A56.

31. Council on Scientific Affairs: Maternal serum α-fetoprotein monitoring. *JAMA* 1982;247:1478-1481.

32. American Society of Human Genetics: Maternal serum alpha-fetoprotein screening programs and quality control for laboratories performing maternal serum and amniotic fluid alpha-fetoprotein assays. *American Journal of Human Genetics* 1987;40:75-82.

33. American Society of Human Genetics: The American Society of Human Genetics Statement on cystic fibrosis screening. *American Journal of Human Genetics* 1990;46:393.

34. National Institutes of Health: Statement from the National Institutes of Health Workshop on population screening for the cystic fibrosis gene. *New England Journal of Medicine* 1990;323:70-71.

35. National Advisory Council for Human Genome Research: Statement on use of DNA testing for presymptomatic identification of cancer risk. *JAMA* 1994;271:785.

36. American Society of Clinical Oncology: Statement of the American Society of Clinical Oncology: Genetic testing for cancer susceptibility, Adopted on February 20, 1996. *Journal of Clinical Oncology* 1996;14:1730-1736.

37. American Society of Human Genetics Ad Hoc Committee: Statement of The American Society of Human Genetics on genetic testing for breast and ovarian cancer predisposition. *American Journal of Human Genetics* 1994;55(5):i-iv.

38. National Breast Cancer Coalition. *Presymptomatic genetic testing for heritable breast cancer risk.* Washington DC, 1995.

39. American College of Medical Genetics: Statement on use of apolipoprotein E testing for Alzheimer disease. *JAMA* 1995;274:1627-1629.

40. National Institute on Aging: Apolipoprotein E genotyping in Alzheimer's disease. *Lancet* 1996;347:1091-1095.

41. Higgs R: *Hazardous to our health? FDA regulation of health care products.* Oakland, Independent Institute; 1995.

42. Merrill RA: Regulation of drugs and devices: An evolution. *Health Affairs* 1994;Summer:46-69.

43. Bogdanich W: False negative. Medical labs, trusted as largely error-free, are far from infallible. *Wall Street Journal* Feb. 2, 1987:1.

44. Bogdanich W: Risk factor. Inaccuracy in testing cholesterol hampers war on heart disease. *Wall Street Journal* Feb. 3, 1987:1.

45. Nash P: Discussion Session I. *Clinical Chemistry* 1992;38:1220-1222.

46. Subcommittee on Technology, Committee on Science, U.S. House of Representatives Hearing on Technological advances in genetics testing: Implications for the future. 1996.

47. U.S.Senate Committee on Labor and Human Resources. Hearing on Advances in Genetics Research and Technologies: Challenges for Public Policy. 1996.

48. American Society of Human Genetics, American College of Medical Genetics: Points to consider: Ethical, legal, and psychosocial implications of genetic testing in children and adolescents. *American Journal of Human Genetics* 1995;57:1233-1241.

49. President's Commission for the Study of Ethical Problems in Medicine and Biomedical and Behavioral Research: *Screening and Counseling for Genetic Conditions.* Washington DC, U.S. Government Printing Office; 1983.

50. American Society of Human Genetics Social Issues Sub-Committee on Familial Disclosure: Professional disclosure of familial genetic information. *American Journal of Human Genetics* 1997;in press.

51. Rothenberg KH: Genetic information and health insurance: State legislative approaches. *Journal of Law, Medicine & Ethics* 1995;23:312-319.

52. Hudson KL, Rothenburg KH, Andrews LB, Kahn MJE, Collins FS: Genetic discrimination and health insurance: An urgent need for reform. *Science* 1995;270:391-393.

53. Rothenberg KH, Fuller B, Rothstein M, et al: Genetic information and the workplace: Legislative approaches and policy challenges. *Science* 1997;275:1755-1757.

54. Eichenwald K: Push for royalties threatens use of Down Syndrome test. *New York Times* May 23, 1997;A1.

55. Clayton EW, Steinberg KK, Khoury MJ, et al: Informed consent for genetic research on stored tissue samples. *JAMA* 1995;274:1786-1792.

56. American College of Medical Genetics: ACMG Statement. Statement on storage and use of genetic materials. *American Journal of Human Genetics* 1995;57:1499-1500.

57. American Society of Human Genetics: ASHG report. Statement on informed consent for genetic research. *American Journal of Human Genetics* 1996;59:471-474.

58. Academy for Clinical Laboratory Physicians and Scientists, et al. Uses of human tissue. August 28, 1996. 1996;draft.

CHAPTER 2. ENSURING THE SAFETY AND EFFECTIVENESS OF NEW GENETIC TESTS

Some predictive genetic tests become available without adequate assessment of their benefits and risks. When this happens, providers and consumers cannot make a fully-informed decision about whether or not to use them. Although extensive use has eventually proved most tests to be of benefit, a few have not proved helpful and were discarded or modified. In the meantime, people were

---

Types of problems encountered in predictive genetic testing.
- Analytical validity. (a) The test does not accurately measure the analyte (substance it is intended to measure). The reason could be contamination (a problem in the polymerase chain reaction (PCR)) or the presence of inhibitors in enzyme assays. (b) The test fails to distinguish trait from disease (Sickledex). (c) The analyte is unstable (galactose-1-phosphate uridyl transferase in screening for galactosemia).
- Clinical validity. (a) The test cannot detect all individuals at risk (cystic fibrosis carrier screening; tests for inherited susceptibility to breast or colon cancer). (b) A positive test result does not always mean disease will develop (apolipoprotein E4 test for Alzheimer disease; breast cancer susceptibility). (c) The test cannot predict the severity of the disease (DNA tests for cystic fibrosis).
- Administration. (a) Specimens are switched (observed occasionally when large numbers of specimens are handled simultaneously as in population-based screening). (b) Specimens are delayed in reaching the laboratory due to batching of specimens before sending; (c) Results are not reported promptly due to weekends and holidays, slow mail, or wrong addresses.
- Pre-test disclosure. Persons being tested (or their parents or legal guardians) are given inadequate information about the test and its implications prior to testing (screening newborns without informing the parents; prenatal screening for neural tube defects or Down syndrome without indicating abortion as an option; presymptomatic testing for Huntington disease without adequate preparation of the at-risk person for coping with the results); failing to inform people about possible difficulties in obtaining insurance and employment, possible risk to others in the family.
- Interpretation of test results. Based on incomplete information provided by the laboratory (a) followup by providers is inappropriate (starting a newborn on special diet for phenylketonuria (PKU) without confirming the screening test result; confusing a positive result for sickle cell trait with the presence of sickle cell disease or vice versa) and/or (b) counseling is inadequate (failing to inform a tested person that a negative test result for susceptibility to common diseases does not rule out the possibility of future disease; failing to tell a pregnant woman that a negative prenatal screening test result does not tell anything about other problems the baby might have).

---

wrongly classified as at-risk and subjected to treatments that, in their case, proved unnecessary or sometimes harmful. Others, who could have benefited from treatment were classified as "normal" and not treated. Harmful effects can be avoided or at least reduced if systematic, well-designed studies to assess a test's safety and effectiveness are undertaken before tests become routinely available and after they are significantly modified. In this chapter, we present criteria for assessing genetic tests prior to routine use, policies for ensuring that the necessary data are collected and, finally, recommendations for review of the data before tests are routinely used.

CRITERIA FOR DEVELOPING GENETIC TESTS

The Task Force strongly holds that the clinical use of a genetic test must be based on evidence that the gene being examined is associated with the disease in question, that the test itself has analytical and clinical validity, and that the test results will be useful to the people being tested. In this section, we first describe these criteria and then consider how adherence to them can be ensured.

Establishing Associations Between a Disease, Genes, and Inherited Mutations

In developing genetic tests, scientists must first be confident that the DNA segments under investigation play a role in the disease in question. These segments might be apparently functionless markers that appear to be spatially linked on a chromosome to a disease-related gene. Linkage is demonstrated when, within families, one form of the marker is found in those with the disease more often than in blood relatives in whom the disease is absent. Because such associations might be due to chance, as was the case for the linkage claimed between bipolar affective disorder and markers on chromosome 11, and between schizophrenia and markers on chromosome 5,[1,2] stringent statistical standards must be satisfied before accepting linkage,[3] and the findings must be confirmed in additional families with the disease. The method has proved successful in locating disease-related genes for Huntington disease, cystic fibrosis, breast cancer, and other disorders.

Further research leads scientists from the linked, functionless marker to a nearby gene suspected of being causally related to the diseases in question. The proof depends on finding mutations in the gene that are only present (in gene dosage sufficient to cause disease) in family members with disease.[a] Further proof that a gene is causally related to disease comes from demonstrating that the protein encoded by the gene is absent, not synthesized in adequate amounts, or manifests a structural or functional aberration that plausibly accounts for symptoms and signs of the disease.

Another approach to identifying a disease-related gene does not depend on linkage but on suspecting that a gene that has been previously identified ("candidate" gene) plays a role in a specific disease. Here too, mutations (in gene dosage sufficient to cause disease) must be found only in those with the disease.

The DNA segments associated with a disease might be functional, common, polymorphic gene variants. Recently, attention has been given to the association between the apolipoprotein E

---

[a] Affected members within one family will each have the same mutation, but in other families different mutations in the same gene can result in disease. There are, for instance, over 600 different mutations in the cystic fibrosis transmembrane regulator gene[4] and over 200 that confer susceptibility to breast cancer in the BRCA1 and BRCA2 genes.[5,6]

polymorphism and Alzheimer disease (AD).[7] A higher proportion of people with apoE4 will develop AD than those with other forms of the polymorphism. Some people with AD, however, will not inherit apoE4 and others with apoE4 will never develop AD;[8] the polymorphism is neither a necessary nor sufficient cause for the disease. In some cases, the polymorphic variants themselves predispose to the disease; in others, the association is spurious (unlikely in the case of apoE4 and AD); and in still others, a marker linked to both the polymorphic gene and the disease-related gene is responsible.[b]

The following criteria must be satisfied before either linked markers or putative disease-related mutations are used as the basis of a genetic test. **The genotypes to be detected by a genetic test must be shown by scientifically valid methods to be associated with the occurrence of a disease. The observations must be independently replicated and subject to peer review.**

Analytical Validity

For DNA-based tests, analytical validity requires establishing the probability that a test will be positive when a particular sequence (analyte) is present (analytical sensitivity) and the probability that the test will be negative when the sequence is absent (analytical specificity).[c] In contrast to DNA-based tests, enzyme and metabolite assays measure continuous variables (enzyme activity or metabolite concentration). One key measure of their analytical validity is accuracy, or the probability that the measured value will be within a predefined range of the true activity or concentration. Another measure of analytical validity is reliability, or the probability of repeatedly getting the same result.

Analytical validation of a new genetic test includes comparing it to the most definitive or "gold standard" method. The first genetic test to be used clinically might, however, be the gold standard; for example, a test that employs sequencing to detect disease-related mutations. In either case, validation includes performing replicate determinations to ensure that a single observation is not spurious, and "blind" testing of coded positive samples (from patients with the disease in whom the alteration is known to be present) and negative samples (from controls). Organizations engaged in new test development should have access to a sufficient number of patient samples to have statistical confidence in the validation. In validating a new test analytically, the laboratory techniques should be as similar as possible to those used when the test will be performed clinically once it is validated.

Analytical sensitivity and specificity of a genetic test must be determined before it is made available in clinical practice.

---

[b] Until recently, it was not clear whether the strong association between the iron-overload disease, hemochromatosis, with polymorphic alleles in the HLA histocompatibility region on chromosome 6 meant that an HLA allele was responsible for the disease or whether it was closely linked to the disease-related gene. As a result of recent research, it is highly likely that a rare allele in the HLA histocompatibility complex is responsible for the disease in most Caucasians. It has a structure resembling other histocompatibility genes. [9]

[c]Gene dosage will also define a positive test result. If detection of carriers is the objective, or the condition being sought is dominant, the test will be positive when one "dose" of a disease-related mutation is present. If detection of those with autosomal recessive conditions is the objective, the test will be positive when two "doses" of a disease related mutation are present.

Clinical Validity

Clinical validation involves establishing several measures of clinical performance including (1) the probability that the test will be positive in people with the disease (clinical sensitivity), (2) the probability that the test will be negative in people without the disease (clinical specificity), and (3) the probability that people with positive test results will get the disease (positive predictive value (PPV))

Parameters of the clinical validity of genetic tests.

		Disease	
		Present	Absent
Test Result	Positive	A	B
	Negative	C	D

A = True positives: those with positive test results who *will* manifest the disease.

B = False positives: those with positive test results who *may* or *may not* have the genetic defect but who *will never* manifest the disease.

C = False negatives: those with negative test results who *will* manifest the disease.

D = True negatives: those with negative test results who will never manifest the disease.

Sensitivity = the probability that the test will be positive in someone who will manifest the condition (**A/A + C**).

Specificity = the probability that the test will be negative in someone who will not manifest the condition (**D/B + D**).

Positive Predictive value = the probability that a person with a positive result will manifest the disease (**A/A + B**).

Negative predictive value = the probability that a person with a negative result will not manifest the disease (**D/C + D**).

---

and that people with negative results will not get the disease (negative predictive value). Predictive value depends on the prevalence of the disease in the group or population being studied, as well as on the clinical sensitivity and specificity of the test.

Two intrinsic features of genetic diseases, heterogeneity and penetrance, affect clinical validity.

Heterogeneity. The same genetic disease might result from the presence (in the necessary gene dosage) of any of several different variants (alleles) of the same gene (allelic diversity) or of different genes (locus heterogeneity). With current technology, all disease-related alleles cannot always be identified, particularly when there are many of them, which is often the case. This failure to detect all disease-related mutations reduces a test's clinical sensitivity.

Penetrance. The probability that disease will appear when a disease-related genotype is present is the penetrance of the genotype. When penetrance is incomplete, PPV is reduced. Penetrance is incomplete when other genetic or environmental factors must be present. In high-risk breast cancer families, 10 to 15 percent of women with inherited susceptibility mutations of the BRCA1 gene will never develop breast cancer. Environmental factors and possibly other inherited factors are required as well. In women without a family history of breast cancer, the penetrance of a BRCA1 or BRCA2 mutation is even lower.[10] Alleles at other gene loci and similar environments are more likely to be shared by relatives than by people in the general population.

Sensitivity can be estimated by determining the proportion of all known (symptomatic) patients with the disease in whom the test is positive. For direct DNA tests for inherited mutations whose causal role has been established, the mutation is not an effect of the disease. Therefore, determining the sensitivity in symptomatic people is a valid measure of its sensitivity among asymptomatic people. This might not be the case for tests of enzyme activity or metabolite concentration, however. They might be "effects" rather than "causes." Moreover, substances might interfere with their detection. Consequently, validation entails performing the test in healthy individuals. This can be accomplished in pilot screening programs discussed further in chapter 3.

PPV can be estimated by comparing the frequency of positive test results in *healthy* people younger than the age at which the disease first manifests to their frequency in *healthy* people who exceed the age by which the disease usually appears. Subtracting the second frequency from the first gives a crude estimate of penetrance. This method does not take into consideration differences in mortality rates from competing causes. A more definitive but time-consuming method is prospective followup of people tested in a pilot study. Having a treatment available that *might* prevent symptoms of the disease complicates such a study. If all people with positive tests results are treated, it will be impossible to determine whether the failure of the disease to manifest is due to incomplete penetrance or the effects of the intervention. A randomized controlled trial, in which only half of the subjects at risk are treated, can help establish the efficacy of the intervention and the penetrance of the inherited mutation.

Prospective studies can take years. If widespread use of a genetic test is withheld until PPV is fully determined, manufacturers and commercial laboratories could be inhibited from developing tests and, consequently, people denied the benefits that might accrue as a result of being tested. Later in this chapter we discuss solutions to this problem.

Parameters of clinical validity will depend in part on the group or population in which the test will be used. For instance, the frequency of disease-related alleles might differ between ethnic groups, making it difficult if not impossible to extrapolate test sensitivity from one group to another. This is the case for cystic fibrosis and breast cancer in which certain alleles can predominate in one ethnic group or geographical area but not in others.[11,12] Penetrance can also differ among ethnic groups. The prevalence of allele frequencies will have a marked effect on PPV; the greater the prevalence, the higher the PPV. Age will also affect allele prevalence; in a population older than the age at which the disease usually causes death, the allele frequency will be lower than in a younger population. For all these reasons, validation studies should be conducted in a group representative of the one in which the test is intended for clinical use.

When tests developed for one purpose are used for another, there is no assurance that the sensitivity or PPV will be the same. The maternal serum alpha-fetoprotein (MSAFP) test was formally validated and approved by the Food and Drug Administration (FDA) as a screening test for open fetal neural tube defects. When it was subsequently discovered that a low MSAFP could predict an increased probability of Down syndrome in the fetus, it quickly was used for this purpose without systematic formal validation. The sensitivity and PPV of the MSAFP test for Down syndrome and other chromosome abnormalities are lower than for neural tube defects.[13] Data on a particular intended use of a test is needed before that use becomes generally accepted clinical practice.[d]

The three following criteria help ensure that appropriate data on the clinical validity of genetic tests will be collected during the developmental stages.

- **Data to establish the clinical validity of genetic tests (clinical sensitivity, specificity, and predictive value) must be collected under investigative protocols.**
- **In clinical validation, the study sample must be drawn from a group of subjects representative of the population for whom the test is intended.**
- **Formal validation for each intended use of a genetic test is needed.**

Clinical Utility

The development of tests to predict future disease often precedes the development of interventions to prevent, ameliorate, or cure that disease in those born with genotypes that increase the risk of disease. Even during this therapeutic gap, benefits might accrue from testing as discussed in chapter 1, such as the ability to avoid the conception or birth of an affected child, reduction of uncertainty and, in those with negative results, escape from frequent monitoring for signs of disease or prophylactic surgery and fear of insurance or employment discrimination. In the absence, however, of definitive interventions for improving outcomes in those with positive test results, the benefits will be limited and not everyone will want to be tested. To improve the benefits of testing, efforts must be made as tests are developed to investigate the safety and effectiveness of new interventions. In the absence of such interventions, studies must be mounted to ensure that testing is beneficial and, particularly, does not inflict psychological harm. The balance of benefits to risks will sometimes depend on how the information is presented and who presents it. These issues are candidates for study. The effect of testing on people with negative, as well as positive results, is important to assess. In high-risk families, people with negative results might have assumed they would be affected and are unprepared to cope with a negative result. They might feel guilt for not having the problem afflicting

---

[d]The Task Force notes that the developer of a genetic test kit, which requires FDA approval before marketing, could maintain in its submission to FDA that the sole intended use of its test is for diagnosis in symptomatic patients. It could then point to a pre-existing (predicate) device and claim that the two were "substantially equivalent." For instance, a developer of a direct DNA test for cystic fibrosis mutations could notify FDA (through a 510(k) notification) that the intended use of its kit is for diagnosis and that it is substantially equivalent to the sweat chloride method, which is standard of care for diagnosing cystic fibrosis. If FDA accepted this substantial equivalence, health care providers could use it for other purposes, such as carrier screening and prenatal diagnosis even though the manufacturer had submitted no information to FDA for those intended uses. The manufacturer cannot, however, include these uses on its label for the test or legally advertise such "off label" uses of its product. FDA does not condone off label use.

their affected relatives.[14] For genetic susceptibility testing, people with negative results might gain the false impression that they have *no* chance of getting the disease and persist in or undertake unhealthful behaviors possibly to their future detriment. Ways should be sought to present information and explanations to minimize inappropriate or erroneous interpretations (see chapter 4). Learning why people who are offered testing decide not to be tested might also help improve understanding of people's perceptions of genetic testing.

The scientists and laboratories developing genetic tests might not have the expertise to explore a number of issues related to communication and counseling. Collaboration with clinical geneticists, genetic counselors, and psychologists can improve the quality of studies looking into these aspects of test development.

Before a genetic test can be generally accepted in clinical practice, data must be collected to demonstrate the benefits and risks that accrue from both positive and negative results.

ENSURING COMPLIANCE WITH CRITERIA

Because of the length of time it can take to establish the appropriateness of a test for clinical use, it is all the more important to ensure the collection of data on safety and effectiveness in the course of test development. At present, no government policy requires the collection of data on clinical validity and utility for all predictive genetic tests under development. Under the Clinical Laboratory Improvement Amendments of 1988 (CLIA), any laboratory providing tests on which clinical decisions are based must demonstrate the tests' analytical validity to outside surveyors, but CLIA has no provision for review of clinical validity or utility. Under the Medical Device Amendments to the Food, Drug, and Cosmetic Act, the safety and effectiveness or substantial equivalence (to devices marketed prior to passage of the Medical Device Amendments in 1976) of clinical diagnostic testing devices, which include genetic testing devices,[e] must be demonstrated prior to marketing. FDA considers clinical validity in assessing safety and effectiveness of clinical laboratory testing devices, but generally not data on followup interventions. The FDA's requirements for demonstrating safety and effectiveness are limited to developers who plan to market genetic testing kits.[f] The FDA has acknowledged to the Task Force that it has the authority to regulate

---

[e]"The term 'device'...means an instrument, apparatus, implement, machine, contrivance, implant, in vitro reagent, or other similar or related article which is... intended for use in the diagnosis of disease or other conditions, or in the cure, mitigation, treatment, or prevention of disease..."(21 U.S.C. 321(h))

[f]The FDA is currently proposing that manufacturers of analyte specific reagents (ASRs) must register with the FDA. In a written response to FDA, a majority of the Task Force held that the FDA's proposal does not adequately protect the public in the development of predictive genetic tests (see appendix 2 for full text). Manufacturers of kits that incorporate ASRs must seek FDA clearance or approval before the test can be promoted for diagnostic use. FDA's review of the kit will include a determination of clinical validity. The FDA proposal does not, however, require demonstration of clinical validity of commercial or other laboratories that incorporate purchased ASRs into tests they market as clinical laboratory services (home brews) rather than kits, or who make their own ASRs.

genetic tests marketed as services but is not doing so. (Personal communications from D. Bruce Burlington, M.D. Director, Center for Devices and Radiological Health, FDA, April 3, 1996) Organizations applying for Federal grants to develop genetic tests must submit their research proposals to peer review "study sections." Institutional review boards (IRBs) must also approve

---

IRB and FDA approval in genetic test development. In the survey of genetic testing organizations conducted for the Task Force, of the 43 biotechnology companies developing or offering genetic tests, only 53.5% had ever submitted a protocol to an IRB and only 30.2% had ever contacted FDA. Of the 215 not-for-profit organizations developing genetic tests (most of which are publicly supported), 60.9% had ever submitted to an IRB and only 7.9% had ever contacted FDA. For organizations of both types using home brews for testing, 73.4% had ever submitted to an IRB and 15.6% had ever contacted FDA (see table 4, appendix 3).

---

protocols submitted to study sections for Federal funding. Many genetic tests, particularly for common disorders, are being developed without Federal funds for research and are not, therefore, subject to peer review. Under FDA regulations, organizations developing new medical devices must have their investigational protocols approved by an IRB. If test results are reported for clinical use and there is no confirmatory test available, the developer must comply with FDA's Investigational Device Exemption regulations. The FDA has not enforced this regulation for developers planning to market tests as services. A number of organizations developing or offering genetic tests, including those who market their own tests (home brews), have never submitted a protocol to an IRB or contacted FDA.

Institutional Review Board (IRB) Review

Considering the structures for external review of research in the U.S. today, the Task Force is of the opinion that IRBs are the most appropriate organizations to consider whether the scientific merit of protocols for the development of genetic tests warrants the risk, however minimal, to subjects participating in the research.

Protocols for the development of genetic tests that can be used predictively must receive the approval of an institutional review board (IRB) when subject identifiers are retained and when the intention is to make the test readily available for clinical use, i.e., to market the test. IRB review should consider the adequacy of the protocol for: (a) the protection of human subjects involved in the study, and (b) the collection of data on analytical and clinical validity, and data on the test's utility for individuals who are tested. IRB review is not needed for minor changes in tests (e.g., detection of additional mutations) as long as the original test was reviewed by an IRB. IRBs may request notification of such changes, however.

Tests under development must be conducted in CLIA-certified laboratories if the results will be reported to patients or their providers.

Health department laboratories or other public agencies developing new genetic tests that satisfy these conditions must also submit protocols to properly-constituted IRBs.

In the early stages of test development, analytical validity and clinical sensitivity can be established using specimens from which identifiers have been removed. (For clinical sensitivity, it need only be known whether the specimen came from someone with disease; identity need not be known.) Using specimens stripped of identifiers prevents contacting subjects. In this case, IRB approval is not needed, although some IRBs might want to know of such studies.[15] It would be more problematic to remove identifiers (anonymizing) in an attempt to estimate PPV. Positive test results on specimens from people who were healthy at the time the specimen was collected need to be followed up to see if disease subsequently appeared. Plans to contact the people or examine their medical records require IRB review and approval. Although recontact might be needed to establish PPV, it might not be appropriate to inform people of results. Informing of results would be appropriate only at a stage when the clinical validity of the test has been fairly well established and when some benefit accrues to the subject from knowing the result. Protocols should spell out what subjects will be told when they are invited to participate in the study, if and under what circumstances they will be recontacted and how recontact will be made, and under what circumstances they will be given results.

The Task Force recognizes that the development of genetic tests is an iterative process; methodological changes to improve sensitivity and, perhaps, specificity, will be made. As already indicated, such changes do not require submission of new protocols to an IRB. Changes in the population or group being tested in the developmental stage, or in the purposes of testing should be submitted for IRB review, with appropriate justification, as an amendment to the original protocol.

Is Review of the Scientific Merit of Genetic Test Protocols Within the Purview of IRBs? Institutional review boards were established to protect human subjects from the risks of participating in research.[g] Genetic test development entails a quest for information in order to advance medical

---

Risks from research intended to develop new predictive genetic tests. The physical risks of test development are usually negligible, involving either a venipuncture, or even less invasively, buccal scraping or collection of hair roots. There can, however, be other risks. Subjects who give consent to the use of their specimen with retention of identifiers would be ethically and legally obliged to say they had been tested and to give the results, if they knew them, when queried about testing (e.g., in purchasing insurance or after being hired for a new job). As a result, subjects could be denied insurance or employment. If they did not know the results, the third party could obtain them from the investigator's records unless the investigator held a certificate of confidentiality. [17]

The use of all or part of a specimen from which all identifiers are removed might unknowingly deny subjects future benefit from use of the specimen unless they are informed. The retention of ethnic or other data with the specimen, even when individual identifiers are removed, might permit uses that subjects would not approve of if they were given the opportunity (e.g., developing genetic tests targeted to certain groups).[17]

---

[g] The Office of the Protection from Research Risks (OPRR) defines research as "a systematic investigation, including research development, testing and evaluation, designed to develop or contribute to generalizable knowledge." (45 CFR 46.102(d)). The Belmont Report, which was the basis for much subsequent

practice and clearly falls under the rubric of research. Any research involving humans entails some risk. Even for research in which the risk to subjects is minimal, the risk should not be taken unless the research has scientific merit. OPRR has commented "if a research project is so methodologically flawed that little or no reliable information will result, it is unethical to put subjects at risk *or even to*

A partial checklist for assessing the scientific merit of protocols for genetic test development.	**A partial checklist for assessing risks of genetic test development.**
• Has the association between the gene locus and disease been confirmed? If not, how will the protocol confirm it? • Has the developer demonstrated the analytical validity of the test or will it be established in the protocol? • Is the proposed study group representative of the group or population for which the test is intended in clinical use? • How will the developer estimate the clinical validity (sensitivity, specificity, PPV) of the test? • Have the interventions available to those who have positive test results been proven to be safe and effective? If not, what plans does the developer have for following subjects with positive test results? • Does the developer have plans for assessing the psychological effects of testing?	• If specimens will be used anonymously, a) Was the purpose for which the specimens were originally collected consistent with their use for genetic test development? b) Did (or will) subjects consent to anonymization for subsequent use? • Will use of the specimen significantly reduce the remaining amount? • If identifiers are being retained, a) Will subjects' consents be obtained? b) What procedures are proposed for recontact or notification? c) If subjects will be informed of the results (i) have they been told this in advance? and (ii) have they been apprised of the implications? d) Who will have access to the results? e) Are subjects' consents required before release of results? f) How will confidentiality of results be ensured? • Where and for how long will specimens be stored? • If specimens will be retained, (a) Who will have access to specimens? and (b) Will subjects' consents for release of specimens be obtained?

Federal policy on protection of human subjects, notes that in situations in which research and practice are carried on together, "that activity should undergo review for the protection of human subjects."[16] Thus a protocol for validating a new genetic test in which the results were given to subjects or their physicians, perhaps for them to base a clinical decision on, would still be considered research. FDA draws a distinction between devices labeled (1) "for research use only," which may not be used in diagnostic procedures or in clinical studies, and (2) "for investigational use only," which are used to establish the performance properties of the device and for which results may or may not be reported. FDA requires that devices "for investigational use only" be subject to IRB oversight.

inconvenience them through participation in such a study" (emphasis added).[18(p. 4-1)] As part of their duty to protect, IRBs must assess the scientific merit of protocols. Most protocols for the development of genetic tests will have scientific merit if they satisfy the criteria enumerated above. In order to protect human subjects in the development of genetic tests, IRBs must recognize the risks posed by genetic test development and determine that investigators have taken adequate steps to apprise subjects of these risks and reduce the chance of harm from those risks.[19,20]

Improving IRB's Ability to Review Genetic Test Protocols. The Task Force recognizes that assistance to IRBs in assessing genetic testing protocols would be helpful. After receiving considerable comment, the Task Force rejected creation of a National Genetics Board (NGB) that could review protocols requiring stringent scrutiny or set general guidelines for IRB review and provide consultation to IRBs on request.[21] An NGB would add another layer of bureaucracy and further delay approval of research protocols.

The Task Force recommends that the Office of Protection of Human Subjects from Research Risks (OPRR) develop guidelines to assist IRBs in reviewing genetic testing protocols. The proposed Secretary's Advisory Committee should work with OPRR to accomplish this task. OPRR and the Advisory Committee should consider how they can be kept apprised of protocols being submitted, in order for them to formulate relevant advice. One possibility is that IRBs submit a one page summary of each genetic testing protocol to OPRR or the group that is developing guidance. The information could include the name of the investigator and his/her institution, the disease for which the test is being developed, intended use, method proposed, and population being studied. Based on these brief reports, the group developing guidance could request protocols for further study but would have no authority to interfere with local IRB review. The protocols would help the group develop general guidance criteria for local IRBs in future reviews.

In developing guidelines for IRBs, OPRR should focus first on tests under development that require stringent scrutiny. **The proposed Secretary's Advisory Committee or its designate, in cooperation with OPRR, should establish criteria for stringent scrutiny.** In addition to the three criteria mentioned in chapter 1--(1) tests that have the ability to predict future disease in healthy or apparently healthy people; (2) tests that are likely to be used for predictive purposes; and (3) tests for which no independent confirmation is available--others should be considered. These criteria include: (4) tests likely to have low sensitivity (due to genetic heterogeneity) and low positive predictive value (due to incomplete penetrance); (5) tests for which no intervention is available or proven to be effective in those with positive test results; (6) tests for disorders of high prevalence; (7) tests likely to be used for screening; and (8) tests likely to be used selectively in ethnic groups with higher incidence or prevalence of the disorder.[h]

Conflict of Interest. **The Task Force recommends strenuous efforts by all IRBs (commercial and academic) to avoid conflicts of interest, or the appearance of conflicts of interest, when reviewing specific protocols for genetic testing. OPRR should consider more stringent standards for all types of IRBs for avoiding conflict of interest situations.** Situations

---

[h]In considering whether a test needs stringent scrutiny, OPRR and the Proposed Secretary's Advisory Committee could assign a score to each of the characteristics they think is important and define tests needing stringent scrutiny tests as all those above a certain score. Alternatively, they could devise an algorithm for assessing how a test meets these characteristics.

in which a close colleague of the investigator is also the local expert on genetic testing pose a difficult problem for university IRBs. Such colleagues should recuse themselves and, if necessary, the IRB should obtain outside consultation. Another difficult situation arises in small companies in which development of a test is crucial to the company's success. Companies should consider using independent IRBs to avoid the appearance of a conflict of interest.

Enforcement. As previously mentioned, organizations that are developing genetic test kits would be expected to submit their investigative protocols to IRBs. FDA can decline to consider applications containing data from clinical investigations that have not been approved by an IRB. Organizations using Federal research funds for genetic test development are also required to obtain IRB approval. Tests developed without Federal funds, either commercially, in academic clinical laboratories, or in some health departments, are not, at the moment, in legal jeopardy if they do not obtain IRB approval.[i] **Testing organizations should comply voluntarily with obtaining IRB approval of genetic test protocols.** Other options the Task Force considered for enforcing the requirement for IRB approval included ensuring that: (1) the FDA use its authority to require all test developers, regardless of whether they plan to market tests as services or kits, to submit protocols to IRBs, (2) third-party payers refuse to reimburse for a genetic test unless the developer can show that it conducted validation/utility studies under an IRB-approved protocol,[j] (3) clinical laboratory surveyors (see chapter 3) confirm that laboratories have received IRB approval of the new genetic tests they developed, and (4) Congress enacts legislation requiring submission of all research protocols, regardless of support, to an IRB.

Data Collection

Investigators given IRB approval for their genetic test protocols have the primary responsibility for data collection under the protocols. To expedite data collection, collaborative efforts will often be needed. For uncommon diseases, a single investigator will seldom have a sufficient number of specimens that contain all or most possible disease-related mutations. Collaboration with investigators who can provide independent sets of specimens or patients increases the likelihood that more mutations will be represented and lends greater statistical confidence to assessments of validity. In assessing tests for susceptibility mutations, having a wider range of

---

[i]New York State requires that investigational clinical laboratory tests receive IRB review. In addition, the Department of Health must approve the investigational use. (State of New York, Department of Health, Genetic Testing Quality Assurance Program: Generally Accepted and Investigational Tests and Procedures, undated.)

[j] P. John Seward, Executive Vice President of the American Medical Association commented on these first two recommendations as they appeared in the Federal Register:[21(p. 4541)] "The suggestion that the FDA ensure that organizations developing new genetic tests submit protocols to local institution review boards (IRBs) is sensible and conforms with existing practice in better scientific institutions. The process would not require centralization and cross-reporting, and could achieve a great deal in the way of controlling wayward test-developers. Also, Medicare, Medicaid and the Civilian Health and Medical Program of the Armed Services (CHAMPUS) would certainly be within their rights to refuse reimbursement for genetic tests which had not been, and were not in the process of being, validated; and can--indeed, already do--insist that labs be qualified." (Communication from Dr. Seward to Task Force, March 11, 1997.)

patients of various ages obtained from different sources will shorten the time to getting a reliable estimate of PPV. Collaboration will also expedite assessing the safety and effectiveness of interventions in people with positive test results that might be included in protocols to measure test validity.

In other research fields, collaborative research has sometimes been delayed by the necessity of obtaining the approval of each collaborating institution's IRB under current regulations.[22] **OPRR, with input from the proposed Secretary's Advisory Committee on genetic testing, should streamline the requirements for IRB review of multicenter collaborative protocols for genetic test development in order to reduce costs and get the studies quickly underway. The Task force calls on Federal agencies, particularly NIH and the Centers for Disease Control and Prevention (CDC) to support consortia and other collaborative efforts to facilitate collection of data on the safety and effectiveness of new genetic tests. CDC should play a coordinating role in data gathering and should be allocated sufficient funds for this purpose. In any sharing or pooling of data, confidentiality of the subject source of the data must be strictly maintained.**

There is, for instance, no reason why a central coordinating agency needs to know the names of subjects with positive or negative test results.

Because it has programs in place, CDC's role is particularly suited to collecting data in healthy populations (e.g., on disease-related allele frequencies). CDC could also establish procedures for tracking healthy individuals with positive test results, as well as those diagnosed with inherited disorders, to learn more about test validity, the natural history of such disorders, and the safety and effectiveness of interventions. The collection of this data should be undertaken in cooperation with test developers, health care providers, and consultants in genetics and other relevant specialties.

CDC could also function as a repository of data submitted to it by organizations competing in the development of a specific test who might not want to collaborate and share data. Respecting proprietary rights, CDC could periodically and confidentially assess the pooled data for validity and utility of the test, providing feedback to the participants on the overall findings.

The Task Force welcomes recent CDC initiatives to expand its population-based surveillance systems in order to provide data on the validity of genetic tests and post-test interventions, and to conduct epidemiologic studies to learn more about test validity, the natural history of genetic disorders, and the safety and effectiveness of interventions. These efforts should be in collaboration with other Federal and State agencies and private organizations.

The Need for Post-market Surveillance

Compliance with all of the criteria for assessment of genetic test validity and utility might be difficult. It can take years to determine whether a disease will appear in healthy people with positive test results or to establish whether an intervention is safe and effective in preventing or ameliorating the disease in question. The Task Force is concerned that the requirements for prolonged data collection might inhibit test development, especially if commercial firms cannot secure a profit until a test is recognized as being suitable for clinical use.[k] Adoption of the recommendations in the

---

[k]FDA regulations allow developers to recover costs during the investigation of medical devices, but not secure a profit. FDA also prohibits them from promoting the device for diagnostic use. As FDA does not now regulate genetic tests planned for marketing as services, developers of genetic testing services are under no price

35

following section would facilitate rapid introduction with collection of the data necessary for assessing validity and utility.

The Task Force recognizes that assessing the validity and utility of some genetic tests will take a long time. When preliminary data indicate a test is likely to have validity and utility, the test should be approved for marketing (see below) but developers must continue to collect data until more definitive answers are obtained. Options for encouraging collection of the requisite data include the following.

(1) Voluntary collection of data by developers after their tests enter clinical use. They would have to develop a reporting mechanism to correlate test results with subsequent occurrence of disease. CDC could coordinate collection of this data from different testing laboratories as discussed above.

(2) Reimbursement for, or coverage of, tests by third-party payers, including government programs, such as Medicare, Medicaid, CHAMPUS, and managed care organizations, during investigative stages in which data are being collected.[23]

(3) Conditional premarket approval by the FDA of genetic test kits. When FDA considers it likely that the test will prove to make an important contribution to the prevention or management of the disorder, it should grant conditional premarket approval when a developer requests it. (FDA frequently clears or approves products for a limited-indication use with the requirement for postmarket studies or the expectation that claims may be extended as sufficient evidence accumulates.) Tests deemed to require stringent scrutiny should be included. In return for conditional approval, developers could include a profit markup in the price. They could promote the test but would have to indicate that the safety and effectiveness of the test were still under investigation. Informed consent would be needed, but as noted in chapter 1, informed consent for predictive genetic tests is a Task Force principle for many genetic tests in clinical use. Developers of kits would continue to collect and periodically present data to the FDA until such time as the agency gives unconditional approval for marketing. FDA should be required to review the data periodically and decide at each point whether to grant unconditional approval, continue data collection under conditional approval, or revoke conditional approval.

EVIDENCE-BASED ENTRY OF NEW GENETIC TESTS INTO CLINICAL PRACTICE

Although IRBs receive a final report of investigative studies they have approved, they have no responsibility to assess the quality of the data or whether it supports the conclusions of the investigators. Considering the potential widespread use of some genetic tests and their importance, **test developers must submit their validation and clinical utility data to internal as well as independent external review. In addition, test developers should provide information to professional organizations and others in order to permit informed decisions about routine use.** External review should take place after data have been collected and near the point when developers believe their tests are ready for clinical use not exclusively under investigative protocols. The Task Force recognizes that not all new genetic tests are in need of such review. **The proposed**

---

constraints in the developmental stages. Moreover, they can decide themselves when a test is marketable.

Secretary's Advisory Committee should suggest criteria for external review, and recommend means of ensuring that review of tests requiring stringent scrutiny will take place. To accomplish the latter, the cooperation of various government and nongovernment groups to conduct reviews must be secured, as well as funds to support the reviews. Review should take place at the local, as well as national level. A wide range of stakeholders should participate in reviews.

Review panels could become enmeshed in endless debate if they attempt to set cutpoints for sensitivity and PPV; these should vary depending on the particular test, its use, options for treatment, and other factors. Even for a particular test, reasonable people will differ on how much test uncertainty they can tolerate.[24,25] It is more important for external reviewers to ensure that the data have been appropriately collected and analyzed than to attempt to set cutpoints. They should also review proposed informational material to make sure the data are interpreted correctly and that test limitations (such as imperfect sensitivity and PPV) are indicated. Review panels could suggest those groups that should consider using the test and those that should not.

The iterative nature of test development makes it likely that methodological improvements will be made in predictive genetic tests. If such changes are made prior to external review, developers can use the data collected before the changes as a "baseline" to demonstrate the improvements, e.g., in test sensitivity. If a test has already been externally reviewed, and the methodological changes alter the target groups, the purposes of testing, or other significant aspects, re-review should be considered by the proposed Secretary's Advisory Committee or other organizations.

Local Review

The first level of local review is by the clinical laboratory that plans to make the test available for clinical use (see chapter 3). In addition, independent local review is also needed, particularly to assess clinical validity and utility. **The Task Force strongly suggests that any organization in which tests are developed conduct a structured review of the analytic and clinical validity and utility of new genetic tests before marketing them or otherwise making them available for clinical use. This structured review should be conducted by those not actually involved in developing the test and collecting the data.** Some medical centers have standing committees that review tests proposed to be offered in the institution's clinical laboratories that could serve

Local review of new genetic tests. In the Department of Laboratory Medicine and Pathology at Mayo Clinic, new test proposals require peer review by members of the Department and by clinical colleagues. First, a Test Abstract (which includes background information, medical use, clinical pathologic correlations, method, likely interpretations of results, cautions, and references) is distributed to consultants and laboratory supervisors within the Department with an invitation for comments. Second, clinicians who would potentially use the test are asked to review the proposal and supporting data. Third, the entire Test Proposal Packet is reviewed by colleagues in the same Division as the proposing laboratory (e.g., Division of Laboratory Genetics). Outcomes of the Division review can be approval of the test, suggestions for modifications to the test or its utilization, or a requirement for additional method validation. Final review and approval of the Test Proposal Packet is by the Chair of the Department of Laboratory Medicine and Pathology.-- Communication to the Task Force from Karen Snow, Division of Laboratory Genetics, Mayo Clinic, July 22, 1997.

this function. For commercial organizations, a unit within the company, but independent of the laboratory that is actually developing the test, should review the data.

National Review

Current legal requirements that genetic tests be reviewed prior to their clinical use apply only to tests marketed as kits, which require premarket approval by FDA. Even if FDA were to include in its purview genetic tests marketed as services, its review would not address all issues of concern to the Task Force. First, FDA does not generally assess safety and effectiveness of a laboratory test in terms of its ability to improve outcomes of those undergoing testing. Second, FDA generally limits its review to the intended uses of a test claimed by the test's sponsor in its premarket notification. Except when it restricts use of a test to specified purposes, which it has the authority to do, FDA does not exert its power to prevent a test marketed for one intended use to be used for other purposes. This is one reason why the Task Force urges developers to undertake formal validation for each intended use of a genetic test.

To improve FDA perspectives on genetic testing and related issues, the Task Force recommends that FDA bring together consultants on genetic testing either from existing panels or by constructing a new panel to provide guidance to FDA on the classification levels needed for genetic testing devices with single or multiple intended uses. Not all devices may require comparable types of review. In conjunction with the proposed Secretary's Advisory Committee considering stringent scrutiny of genetic tests, these consultants should identify aspects of genetic testing that affect the classification level.

Although no other legally-required mechanisms currently exist, other reviews can have a profound influence on providers' decisions to use, or not use, new medical technologies. Examples are: statements of professional societies, consensus development panels, and ratings by the U.S. Preventive Services Task Force.[26] The decision of health insurers on whether a specific genetic test will be included in their benefits or reimbursement packages can also influence use and will be based on the insurers' own reviews (M Schoonmaker, submitted for publication) or other external reviews. A recent consensus development panel on cystic fibrosis carrier screening provides an example of national external review.[4]

Review organizations could select the tests in the greatest need of review by using the criteria for stringent scrutiny to be developed by the proposed Secretary's Advisory Committee. The reviews would be based primarily on data collected during the test development stage or during the proposed conditional premarket approval stage. Depending on how interest in a test expands, on technological changes, and on other considerations, reviewers could periodically reassess the test as the Preventive Services Task Force does for the interventions it reviews.[26]

REFERENCES

1. Risch N, Botstein D: A manic depressive history. *Nature Genetics* 1996;12:351-353.

2. Schwab SG, Albus M, Hallmayer J, et al: Evaluation of a susceptibility gene for schizophrenia on chromosome 6p by multipoint affected sib-pair linkage analysis. *Nature Genetics* 1995;11:325-327.

3. Lander E, Kruglyak L: Genetic dissection of complex traits: Guidelines for interpreting and reporting linkage results. *Nature Genetics* 1996;11:241-247.

4. Genetic testing for cystic fibrosis: NIH Consensus Statement, 1997:15(4)1-37.

5. Healy B: BRCA genes--Bookmaking, fortunetelling, and medical care. *New England Journal of Medicine* 1997;336:1448-1449.

6. Friend S, Borresen AL, Brody L, et al: Breast cancer information on the web. *Nature Genetics* 1995;11:238-239.

7. Morrison-Bogorad M, Phelps C, Buckholtz N: Alzheimer disease research comes of age. The pace accelerates. *JAMA* 1997;277:837-840.

8. Seshadri S, Drachman DA, Lippa CF: Apolipoprotein E e4 allele and the lifetime risk of Alzheimer's disease. What physicians know, and what they should know. *Archives of Neurology* 1995;52:1074-1079.

9. Feder JN, Gnirke A, Thomas W, et al: A novel MHC class I-like gene is mutated in patients with hereditary haemochromatosis. *Nature Genetics* 1996;13:399-408.

10. Struewing JP, Hartge P, Wacholder S, et al: The risk of cancer associated with specific mutations of BRCA1 and BRCA2 among Ashkenazi Jews. *New England Journal of Medicine* 1997;336:1401-1408.

11. Cutting G: Cystic fibrosis. in Rimoin DL, Connor JM, Pyeritz RE (eds): *Principles and Practice of Medical Genetics.* London, Churchill Livingstone; 1996.

12. Szabo CI, King M: Invited editorial: Population genetics of BRCA1 and BRCA2. *American Journal of Human Genetics* 1997;60:1013-1020.

13. American College of Obstetricians and Gynecologists: Maternal serum screening. *ACOG Educational Bulletin* 1996;228:1-9.

14. Wexler NS: The Tiresias complex: Huntington's disease as a paradign of testing for late-onset disorders. *FASEB Journal* 1992;6:2820-2835.

15. Clayton EW, Steinberg KK, Khoury MJ, et al: Informed consent for genetic research on stored tissue samples. *JAMA* 1995;274:1786-1792.

16. The National Commission for the Protection of Human Subjects of Biomedical and Behavioral Research: The Belmont Report. Ethical principles and guidelines for the protection of human subjects of research. *OPRR Reports* April 18, 1979:2-8.

17. Holtzman NA, Andrews LB: Ethical and legal issues in genetic epidemiology. *Epidemiologic Reviews* 1997;in press.

18. Office of Protection from Research Risks: *Protecting Human Research Subjects. Institutional Review Board Guidebook.* Washington DC, U.S. Government Printing Office; 1993.

19. Glass KC, Weijer C, Palmour RM, Shapiro SH, Lemmens TM, Lebacqz K: Structuring the review of human genetics protocols: Gene localization and identification studies. *IRB* 1996;18:1-9.

20. Glass KC, Weijer C, Palmour RM, Lemmens TM, Shapiro SH: Structuring the review of human genetics protocols part II: Diagnostic and screening studies. *IRB* 1997;19(3):1-11; 19(4):13. *Research* 1997;in press.

21. National Institutes of Health: Proposed recommendations of the Task Force on Genetic Testing; Notice of meeting and request for comment. *Federal Register* 1997;62:4539-4547.

22. Levine RJ: Ethics and epidemiology. in Coughlin SS, Beauchamp TL (eds): New York, Oxford University Press; 1996:257-273.

23. Gleeson S: Blue Cross and Blue Shield Association initiatives in technology assessment. in Gelijns AC, Dawkins HV (eds): *Medical Innovation at the Crossroads Vol IV: Adopting New Medical Technology.* Washington DC, National Academy Press; 1994:96-100.

24. Tambor ES, Bernhardt BA, Chase GA, et al: Offering cystic fibrosis carrier screening to an HMO population: Factors associated with utilization. *American Journal of Human Genetics* 1994;55:626-637.

25. Croyle RT, Dutson DS, Tran VT, Sun Y: Need for certainty and interest in genetic testing. *Women's Health: Research on Gender, Behavior, and Policy* 1995;1:329-339.

26. U.S.Preventive Services Task Force: *Guide to Clinical Preventive Services.* Alexandria, International Medical Publishing, Inc. 1996.

CHAPTER 3. ENSURING THE QUALITY OF LABORATORIES PERFORMING GENETIC TESTS

Over 500 clinical laboratories in the United States perform chromosomal, biochemical, and/or DNA-based tests for genetic diseases (see appendix 3). These laboratories must comply with regulations under the Clinical Laboratory Improvement Amendments of 1988 (CLIA), which include biennial inspection, some proficiency testing, and requirements of the specialty in which the laboratory is certified. Although clinical cytogenetics is a specialty under CLIA, there is no broader genetics specialty and, consequently, no special requirements for laboratories performing DNA-based and other types of genetic tests. No proficiency testing programs in genetics or cytogenetics are required under CLIA. New York State requires any laboratory performing tests on New York residents (even if those laboratories are outside of New York) to participate in its quality assurance programs in DNA-based and biochemical genetics. These programs involve onsite inspection but not formal proficiency testing.[a] A number of organizations have voluntary programs for quality control of genetic tests; they are described later in this chapter. In a survey conducted for the Task Force in early 1995, 11% of biotechnology companies that provide genetic tests and 16% of nonprofit (primarily university-based) molecular (DNA) labs reported that they neither participated in a formal proficiency testing program nor shared samples informally for quality control (see appendix 3). According to the survey, about 15% of laboratories performing clinical DNA-based tests were not registered under CLIA (see chapter 5 for further discussion of this problem).

Although the vast majority of laboratories providing genetic tests perform adequately, the Task Force has two concerns. First, even though most laboratories voluntarily participate in quality programs addressed specifically to genetic tests, they are not required to do so. Consequently, providers and consumers have no assurance that every laboratory performs adequately. Occasionally errors are made. Second, that current requirements under CLIA, with which clinical laboratories must comply, are inadequate to ensure the overall quality of genetic testing because they are not specifically designed for genetic tests and because they do not give sufficient emphasis to pre- and post-analytic phases of testing. Voluntary programs are also lacking on this second point.

In this chapter, we first describe the principles that laboratories should follow in adding new genetic tests to their repertoire. We then consider CLIA's framework for laboratory quality and, in view of gaps in CLIA in the area of genetics, other programs for assessing and improving test performance. We then indicate our concerns about ensuring the quality of the pre- and

---

[a]New York State expects laboratories to establish their own system for monitoring proficiency of these tests. A few other states, including California, are planning oversight of clinical laboratories performing molecular genetic tests.

post-analytic phases of predictive genetic testing. We conclude with brief consideration of the need for a central repository of materials for genetic testing, direct marketing, and international standardization of quality assurance methods.

Errors in Tay-Sachs carrier testing. Although Tay-Sachs carrier screening has led to a marked reduction in the incidence of Tay-Sachs[1] mistakes in testing are sometimes made. "Our [Tay-Sachs] center has been informed of multiple errors, of many different types, associated with laboratory testing. In our own records we have at least eight examples of individuals who have been *identified as carriers* by both private or university laboratories (in various parts of the country) who, for whatever reason, requested retest by our center and were *proven definitively to be noncarriers*. In a similar context, we have identified at least seven or eight instances where individuals were identified as "*inconclusive*" by the laboratories where the initial test was done who were without question *noncarriers* in our facility. In each of the above instances, planned pregnancy intervention testing was about to be carried out, or was, because of the possible at risk status of the family. In several other instances (at least six) individuals with indeterminate results in other centers, who contacted us for further testing, were clearly *proven to be carriers*...I should point out that there have been *15 major litigations* initiated around the issues of negligence in Tay-Sachs testing. (emphasis in original)"--Michael M. Kaback, M.D., Director, International Tay-Sachs Disease Data Collection and Quality Control Program, communication to the Task Force Chair, October 21, 1996.

PRINCIPLES FOR LABORATORIES ADOPTING NEW GENETIC TESTS

No clinical laboratory should offer a genetic test whose clinical validity has not been established, unless it is collecting data on clinical validity under either an IRB-approved protocol or conditional premarket approval agreement with FDA (one of the options presented in chapter 2). The service laboratory should justify and document the basis of decisions to put new tests into service. In accord with the recommendations in chapter 2, a clinical laboratory that develops a genetic test would have to submit its data on analytical and clinical validity to external review before offering the test for clinical practice.[b] If the test has been developed elsewhere, clinical laboratories should carefully review evidence for test validity. If external review by professional societies has led to the publication of indications and guidelines for use, laboratories should adhere to them. Regardless of where the test to be adopted was developed, **clinical laboratory directors are responsible for ensuring the analytic validity of each genetic test their laboratory intends to offer before they make the test available for use in clinical practice (outside of an investigative protocol).** (Methods for assessing analytical validity are summarized in chapter 2.)

---

[b]To avoid submission for external review, a genetic test developer could keep a test in the investigative stage perpetually. This would preclude the developer from ever including a profit in the price of the test unless FDA granted conditional premarket approval as described in chapter 2.

Before routinely offering genetic tests that have been clinically validated, a laboratory must conduct a pilot phase in which it verifies that all steps in the testing process are operating appropriately. In establishing the pilot phase, the laboratory should define endpoints, such as number of tests to be performed,[c] and the procedures to be used to review the findings, including the organizational body that will review them. If the outcome of this review reveals that the laboratory is not as competent as other laboratories in performing the test, or the test does not detect as many people with the genetic alteration as anticipated, the laboratory should not proceed to report patient-specific results without attempting to rectify the problems. If demand is not sufficiently high to be able to maintain a high level of quality, the laboratory should institute special procedures to ensure quality.

During the pilot phase, confidence in the analytical validity of the test can be gained by splitting specimens with another laboratory.[d] This phase can be used to detect and correct problems in test requisitions, specimen transport, data analysis and transcription, reporting of results, and user satisfaction. It can also be used to establish that laboratory staff are capable of deciding whether each requisition for the test meets established criteria, and the staff is capable of performing the tests and interpreting the results correctly. The pilot phase should employ laboratory practices as similar as possible to those planned when the test becomes routinely available.

CLINICAL LABORATORY IMPROVEMENT AMENDMENTS OF 1988 (CLIA)

A statutory framework for ensuring laboratory quality was laid down by Congress in the Clinical Laboratory Improvement Act of 1967 and greatly expanded in the Clinical Laboratory Improvement Amendments of 1988 (CLIA). Any laboratory performing "examination of materials derived from the human body for the purpose of providing information for the diagnosis, prevention, or treatment of any disease or impairment of, or the assessment of the health of, human beings" must comply with CLIA.[2] Implementation of CLIA is the responsibility of the Health Care Financing Administration (HCFA) and the Centers for Disease Control and Prevention (CDC). Under CLIA, these Federal agencies have developed requirements for laboratory quality assurance and control, personnel, patient test-management and, if a proficiency program is not available,

---

[c]The minimum number of specimens should be sufficient for the laboratory to be statistically confident in the clinical sensitivity and specificity of the test.

[d]For example, the American College of Medical Genetics recommends splitting 50 consecutive specimens with an established laboratory in cases of prenatal cytogenetic diagnosis using amniotic fluid. For rare disorders, it may be hard to find a sufficient number of specimens; reliability will be demonstrated by replicate blind testing of as many specimens as possible.

43

interlaboratory comparison of assays. The stringency of these requirements depends on the complexity level and specialty to which tests are assigned. Despite these basic provisions, the Task Force has serious concerns as to whether CLIA adequately assures the quality of genetic tests in clinical use.

History of CLIA. The Clinical Laboratory Improvement Act of 1967 established Federal control over laboratories providing more than 100 tests per year in interstate commerce. Only about 12,000 laboratories reimbursed by Medicare and Medicaid were covered. The Act required the establishment of personnel standards for laboratory directors and other laboratory personnel and quality assurance by laboratory inspection and proficiency testing.

In 1988, the Clinical Laboratory Improvement Amendments (CLIA) were enacted in response to media reports of serious errors and variability in laboratory results, as well as inadequate training and supervision of personnel performing clinical laboratory tests. Serious deficiencies were found in cytology analysis intended to detect cervical cancer (Papanicolaou tests).[3] Public concern had also intensified about the quality of laboratory services provided in physicians' office laboratories. CLIA extended coverage to all laboratories reporting patient-specific clinical test results for purposes other than forensic. In 1997, there are approximately 157,000 CLIA-certified laboratories of which 81,000 are in physicians' offices.

Complexity Ratings

CDC assigns a complexity level to a test according to predetermined criteria. Simple tests are categorized "waived." The remainder are assigned ratings of either "moderate" or "high" complexity. Laboratories performing high complexity tests have more stringent personnel and quality control requirements.

Over 17,000 clinical laboratory tests have been assigned a complexity level.[e] Any test for which CDC has not determined test complexity is considered to be high complexity by default.[f] Any home-brew method, or change in procedure that can affect laboratory performance (sensitivity, specificity, accuracy, precision) falls under the high complexity category until it is rated differently by CDC. Under the rating scheme, a genetic test that can be used predictively might receive a rating of moderate complexity despite the importance of ensuring that the provider and the patient

---

[e]A complete test categorization list can be obtained on the World Wide Web at http://ftp.cdc.gov.

[f]Until a test is assigned a complexity level, "the laboratory (performing it) must have a system for verifying the accuracy and reliability of its test results at least twice a year." (42 CFR sections 493.17, 493.1213 and 493.1217). Moreover, when the laboratory is inspected, its quality control and internal proficiency test system for unrated tests will be examined.

understand the uncertainty of the prediction and the implications for decision-making. Both the creatine phosphokinase test, which can be used as a screening test for Duchenne muscular dystrophy, and alpha-fetoprotein (AFP), which is used as a predictive prenatal test for neural tube defects and Down syndrome, are rated as moderate complexity. Despite multiple uses, a test method gets only

---

Complexity Determinations under CLIA. To be waived, tests must be so simple and accurate as to have negligible risk of error. Laboratories that only have a Certificate of Waiver can only perform waived tests and must follow the manufacturer's instructions. They are not subject to routine inspection. An example of this kind of test is urine analysis by "dipstick."

For non-waived tests, complexity is determined by CDC (in consultation with others), which assigns each test a score of 1, 2, or 3 on each of seven criteria:

(1) The degree of knowledge required to perform the test;
(2) The amount of training and experience required to perform the test;
(3) Necessary preparation of reagents and materials;
(4) The characteristics of operational steps (i.e., whether operational steps are automatically executed or easily controlled, or require close monitoring and/or control);
(5) The nature and availability of calibration, quality control, and proficiency testing materials;
(6) The complexity of troubleshooting and equipment maintenance; and
(7) The degree to which performance of the test depends on interpretation and judgment.

If the total score reaches 12, the test is designated "high complexity." Otherwise, it is "moderate complexity." --Division of Laboratory Systems, Public Health Practice Program Office, CDC.

---

one rating based on the seven criteria (see box entitled Complexity Determinations under CLIA) that reflect the complexity of performing the test. All cytogenetic tests are rated high complexity, which seems appropriate. **The Task Force recommends that tests that can be used for purposes of predicting future disease be given a rating of high complexity.**

CLIA Specialties

Laboratories performing tests of moderate or high complexity must also conform to the requirements of the specialties to which tests are assigned. Laboratories can perform tests only in specialties for which they are certified. Although there is a cytogenetics specialty, there is no genetics specialty.[g] The specialty categories under CLIA are based on traditional laboratory practice; each specialty tends to involve somewhat similar technologies, although this is not the case in all instances. Each analyte is assigned to only one specialty.

---

[g]Medical genetics is recognized as a specialty of medicine by the American Board of Medical Specialties. The American Board of Medical Genetics certifies in cytogenetics, molecular genetics, biochemical genetics, and clinical genetics.

Establishing a specialty for genetics presents a number of problems. For example, specialty designations are administratively linked to Medicare payment specialty designations, and any changes in specialty designations must take this into account. In addition, genetic tests use a wide variety of technologies, some of which are used in other (non-genetic) types of tests. For instance, DNA is the analyte in some tests for predicting genetic susceptibility and also in some tests for infectious agents. Sometimes the same test is used for purposes of genetic prediction (in healthy individuals), genetic diagnosis (in individuals with symptoms), and non-genetic diagnosis or prognosis. For instance, the creatine phosphokinase assay can be used to screen for carriers of muscular dystrophy and affected infants, but it is also used in the diagnosis of myocardial infarction. Despite these problems a genetics specialty is needed.

> **Specialties/Subspecialties under CLIA.** Specialties are microbiology (including subspecialties of bacteriology, mycobacteriology, mycology, parasitology, and virology), immunology (including subspecialties of syphilis serology and general immunology), chemistry (including subspecialties of routine chemistry, endocrinology, toxicology, and urinalysis), hematology, immunohematology, pathology (including subspecialties of cytology, histopathology, and oral pathology), radiobioassay, histocompatibility, and cytogenetics. Petitions for new specialties and subspecialties are made to the Clinical Laboratory Improvement Advisory Committee (CLIAC). CLIAC makes recommendations to CDC, and CDC consults with HCFA and then formulates and implements the specialty/subspecialty designations.

The Task Force welcomes the intention of CDC to create a genetics subcommittee of the Clinical Laboratory Improvement Advisory Committee (CLIAC), which advises on policies under CLIA. The Task Force urges this subcommittee to consider the creation of a specialty of genetics that would encompass all predictive genetic tests that satisfy criteria for stringent scrutiny. If a specialty of genetics is not feasible, the subcommittee should consider a specialty or subspecialty of molecular genetics for DNA/RNA-based tests. In the latter case, it must then address how to ensure the quality of laboratories performing nonDNA/RNA genetic tests. Although DNA-based tests will comprise the largest proportion of predictive tests, for disorders with great allelic diversity, gene product tests might have greater sensitivity than DNA-based tests, at least until technologies that can detect a large proportion of all possible mutations become applicable to clinical testing. **The subcommittee should also consider assigning tests that have widely different uses to more than one specialty.** This will facilitate assigning separate billing and reimbursement codes for each use of a genetic test when the uses are vastly different.

LABORATORY PERSONNEL

Personnel requirements under CLIA, particularly at the level of laboratory director, depend on the specialty and complexity categories to which tests or analytes are assigned. Without a genetics specialty, genetic tests fall into other specialties for which requiring special training in genetics would be superfluous for many of the other tests in those specialties.

<u>Laboratory Director</u>

Under CLIA, a laboratory director must possess a current license as a laboratory director in the state in which the laboratory is located and be either (1) a pathologist; (2) a physician licensed to practice medicine or osteopathy; or (3) a board-certified doctoral scientist (Ph.D.).[h] **The Task Force recommends that for laboratories performing high complexity tests in the proposed specialty of molecular genetics, as well as in biochemical genetics and cytogenetics, personnel serving as directors or technical supervisors must have formal training in human and medical genetics, as documented by holding certification from an organization that assesses knowledge of human and medical genetics as part of its certification process, such as the American Board of Medical Genetics.**

<u>Testing Personnel</u>

CLIA imposes minimal academic qualification requirements for testing personnel.[i] This is reasonable in the area of genetics because most current medical technology training programs include little, if any, exposure to genetics or molecular biology. Several formal training programs for cytogenetics technical staff are available, but there are very few certificate- or diploma-track genetics training programs for technicians or technologists in the U.S. Consequently, most technicians in molecular genetic testing laboratories are trained on the job. Broad backgrounds in genetics are unlikely, as is a familiarity with specialized methodologies involved in molecular genetics testing. **Training programs for laboratory technicians/technologists need more human and medical genetics content than are currently available in the U.S.**

The College of American Pathologists (CAP) specifies a B.S. degree or equivalent in the biological sciences for technologists engaged in genetic testing. Neither CAP nor the American College of Medical Genetics (ACMG) requires personnel to be licensed medical technologists but some States require it. Many States offer a special licensure for cytogenetics technicians; this is a desirable attribute where available. California is presently trying to develop a similar licensing mechanism for molecular genetics technicians. The National Certification Agency is working with the Association of Genetic Technologists to develop certification in genetics. Licensing of technologists performing genetic tests can then be linked to certification. Most clinical molecular genetics laboratories employ technicians with a molecular biology research background.

Biochemical genetic techniques resemble those used in other, more routine, areas of clinical chemistry. For this area, therefore, Federal, State, and professional requirements for clinical

---

[h]As of July 1997, acceptable board certification for physicians includes the American Board of Pathology, and the American Osteopathic Board of Pathology. For doctoral scientists, the American Board of Medical Genetics, the American Board of Medical Microbiology, the American Board of Clinical Chemistry, the American Board of Bioanalysis, the American Board of Medical Laboratory Immunology, the National Registry in Clinical Chemistry, the American Board of Histocompatibility and Immunogenetics, and the American Board of Forensic Toxicology are acceptable under CLIA. Any person who is certified by one of these boards meets the qualification for director regardless of the tests performed in his or her laboratory.

[i]The regulations provide both a phase-in period that allows testing personnel to obtain an associate degree by September 1, 1997, and a grandfather clause for testing personnel who previously qualified or could have qualified as a technologist under 42 CFR 493.1433.

chemistry laboratory personnel are sufficient, as long as the technologists work under a director who is a certified biochemical geneticist.

MONITORING LABORATORY PERFORMANCE

Because laboratories provide services to providers and patients in many States it is clearly more desirable to have a rigorous Federal standard for certification or accreditation than fifty different State standards. Moreover, interstate genetic testing is unavoidable when only one or a few laboratories in the country provide tests. **A national accreditation program for laboratories performing genetic tests, which includes proficiency testing and on-site inspection, is needed to promote standardization across the country.** Such an accreditation program can occur more readily if a genetics specialty were established under CLIA. **Until such time as a genetics specialty is established under CLIA, laboratories performing DNA/RNA-based tests for predictive purposes should choose to voluntarily participate in the CAP molecular pathology program including the CAP/ACMG molecular genetics proficiency testing program.** Laboratories performing genetic tests on analytes not covered in the CAP/ACMG program, such as Tay-Sachs carrier screening and newborn screening, should participate in the available proficiency programs.

Proficiency Testing

Proficiency testing (PT) is mandated by CLIA to externally evaluate the quality of a laboratory's performance. For PT, a laboratory is provided with specimens whose composition of an analyte is known to the supplier but not to the recipient laboratories. They are expected to analyze the specimen the same way they would a patient's specimen. Each laboratory performing moderate or high complexity tests is required to enroll in an approved PT program for all specialties/subspecialties, analytes, or tests for which the laboratory is certified and for which a PT program has been recognized by HCFA. Any laboratory that fails a proficiency test must take corrective action.[j] HCFA takes an educational approach to PT and works with the laboratories that have problems to help improve performance. Sanctions can be applied to those laboratories repeatedly unable to perform satisfactorily. These include suspension of the CLIA certificate to perform that test or specialty. If its certificate is suspended, the laboratory is not eligible for Medicare/Medicaid reimbursement, since such reimbursement requires a CLIA license with no restrictions.

---

[j] CLIA currently requires 3 proficiency challenges per year of 5 analytes each. Failure on 2 challenges in a row or 2 out of 3 triggers an investigation. If the laboratory does not improve, it can be decertified for that particular analyte.

So far, the Department of Health and Human Services has approved 19 PT programs under CLIA. It has not approved proficiency testing programs for genetic tests because such tests do not measure regulated analytes for PT purposes as currently listed in the regulations. New York State and a few regions have cytogenetics PT programs. CAP and ACMG jointly administer PT in

---

Proficiency testing. An example of how proficiency testing can improve the quality of genetics laboratory services is provided by CDC's hemoglobinopathy program. In 1970, the relatively new field of hemoglobinopathy was in chaos. Driven by political pressures to mount programs, many laboratories started to test with no guidelines, no quality control, no proficiency testing, and no central unit to answer questions or resolve problems. The Sickle Cell Branch of NIH funded a National Hemoglobinopathy Laboratory at CDC. Its components included a referral service for diagnosis of problematic specimens, expert consultation, training, evaluation of new methodologies including commercial kits, preparation of standards, and proficiency testing. Proficiency testing was offered originally to any interested laboratory and it was mandatory for centers and clinics funded by NIH. Four specimens were sent four times a year. For laboratories failing testing, CDC analyzed findings in an attempt to pinpoint problems and offer help. Funding was terminated for laboratories that consistently failed to identify proficiency testing materials. In the early rounds of the program, many laboratories had inadequate performance levels. With the guidance given in conjunction with proficiency testing, most laboratories improved their performance on subsequent rounds.

---

cytogenetics, fluorescent in situ hybridization, biochemical genetics, and molecular genetics. In collaboration with the Foundation for Blood Research (FBR), CAP has a PT program for prenatal screening of neural tube defects and Down syndrome. CDC has a PT program for newborn screening tests, including hemoglobinopathies. PT is also available for laboratories worldwide performing Tay-Sachs screening. Responding to a survey conducted for the Task Force in July 1997, CAP, FBR, CDC, and the International Tay-Sachs program reported that most laboratories known to them were participating in their respective programs.[k]

Although genetic tests do not appear on the list of regulated analytes for PT purposes under CLIA, laboratories must establish the accuracy and reliability of a test by methods of their own choosing. This can include participation in one of the voluntary PT programs. As the PT programs mentioned above are not approved by CLIA, no laboratory is obliged to use them and can establish accuracy and reliability by another method, although it must make the data available for onsite inspection under CLIA (see below). If they do participate and do not perform adequately,

---

[k]CAP estimates that about 150 laboratories perform molecular genetics tests of which 127 (85%) participate in the CAP/ACMG PT program. The FBR/CAP program reported that 263 of 268 (98%) laboratories performing prenatal screening for neural tube defects and 253 of 258 (98%) laboratories performing prenatal screening for Down syndrome participated. A similar percentage of the approximately 40 laboratories providing Tay-Sachs carrier screening participated in the International Tay-Sachs Data Collection and Quality Control Program and all of the 60 laboratories providing newborn screening for phenylketonuria participated in CDC's Newborn Screening Quality Assurance program.

laboratories will usually improve performance. If, however, they continue to fail to meet PT criteria, they are not obliged to stop testing as participation is voluntary. A few laboratories participating in the PT programs recently surveyed do not always correctly analyze all PT specimens. According to the Tay-Sachs program, one or two per year do not improve and usually stop testing.

Information collected in conjunction with PT sometimes reveals outliers among laboratories. For instance, a survey conducted by the FBR/CAP prenatal screening PT program found a few laboratories that did not follow established criteria in accepting specimens.

Participation in well-established proficiency testing programs for genetic tests must be required under CLIA once a genetics specialty is established. When no relevant proficiency testing programs exist, laboratories must, whenever possible, participate in inter-laboratory comparison programs and help develop them if none exist in their particular area of testing.

Proficiency testing programs should be broadly based since the number of genetic disorders is very large and the analytical approaches to testing are numerous. It is unlikely that proficiency challenges will ever be constructed for every rare disease or every rare mutation in common diseases for which a given laboratory might test. Because of the similarity of techniques used in biochemical genetics, proficiency in these techniques applied to one or a few analytes is a reasonably good indicator of proficiency in other uses of the technique. CAP/ACMG is expanding the PT offering in molecular genetics to a greater number of disorders in order to get more complete demonstrations of proficiency.

Some laboratories do not follow established criteria for testing. "Sixty-six [of 265 laboratories that participated in the proficiency testing program] offered [prenatal] screening beginning at 14 weeks' gestation or earlier. Four of these offered interpretation at 13 weeks or earlier. Screening for Down syndrome can be feasible at 14 weeks' gestation, but detection of open neural tube defects at this time is poor. At 13 weeks' gestation or earlier, detection of neural tube defects is not possible and Down syndrome detection is poorly defined. Screening at this time in gestation should be discouraged. A few laboratories (8%) offered interpretations of screening after 23 weeks' gestation. The reliability of serum screening for either Down syndrome or open neural tube defects is not known for this time period."[4]

Onsite Inspection

All CLIA-certified laboratories are routinely inspected on a two-year survey cycle[1] by one of three types of organizations: (1) HCFA regional offices and State agencies; (2) private non-profit organizations that have applied for and received deemed status because they provide reasonable assurance that the laboratories they accredit, which enables the laboratory to obtain a CLIA

---

[1]When a complaint is filed against a laboratory, additional inspections may be made. Accrediting organizations and exempt State programs (explained in this section) may conduct complaint investigations. HCFA, however, has the authority to inspect any laboratory that a complaint has been filed against. HCFA considers the nature of the complaint in deciding whether to intervene. The laboratory is responsible for the costs of the investigation in cases in which the complaint is substantiated.

certificate, meet the conditions required by Federal law and regulation;[m] (3) State-exempt licensure programs. States that have programs that license laboratories and provide HCFA with reasonable assurance that their criteria are equivalent to or more stringent than those specified under CLIA can apply for exempt status. So far New York, Oregon, and Washington (state) have exempt status. California, Florida, and Georgia are under review (as of July 1997). Regardless of the organization under whose auspices inspections are conducted, the surveyors are laboratory professionals who are trained to determine compliance with CLIA regulations (or a program that is determined to be equal to or more stringent than CLIA). Even though genetics is not a specialty, surveyors are expected to examine the quality of genetic tests. This should include inspection of the records of how the laboratory performed on genetic PT programs in which it participated voluntarily. It is not clear, however, that all CLIA surveyors currently are sufficiently knowledgeable to assess the performance of molecular genetics laboratories.[n]

CAP has deemed status to conduct inspections in several specialties, but since genetics is not a specialty under CLIA, the CAP program does not have deemed status in genetics. In the CAP genetics program, laboratories who voluntarily (and for a fee) participate in the program are inspected. The surveyors use a checklist covering all aspects of quality assurance and quality control, from specimen accessioning to final sign-out. Compliance with some items on the checklist is optional; for others, compliance is mandatory.[o] Following inspection, the laboratory receives a written report and is expected to respond to CAP in writing regarding correction of any deficiencies in the mandatory categories. In areas in which it does not have deemed status, such as genetics, CAP has no authority to grant accreditation for CLIA purposes.

Making Laboratory Performance Assessments Public

HCFA annually publishes a list ("Laboratory Registry") that identifies all poor performance laboratories, the reason enforcement actions were taken and type of enforcement, and the name of the laboratory director. The Registry is available to the public upon request, and will soon be accessible on the Internet at http://www.hcfa.gov. Survey findings are also available through the Freedom of Information Act, once the laboratory has the opportunity to respond with its Plan of Action. CAP reports PT results for regulated analytes (i.e., those for which CLIA requires PT) to HCFA. It does not report PT results directly to the public because it maintains that PT alone is insufficient to demonstrate laboratory quality. CAP does make accreditation status available through

---

[m]Accrediting organizations receive deemed status for one or more specialties. For instance, the American Society of Histocompatibility and Immunogenetics (ASHI) has been approved only for the specialty of histocompatibility. As a result, any laboratory accredited by ASHI is not subject to routine inspection by either an agent of HCFA or a State survey agency to determine its compliance with the CLIA requirements for histocompatibility. Such labs, however, remain subject to routine inspections by either of those organizations to determine their compliance with CLIA requirements for tests in any other specialty.

[n]Recently, CAP/ACMG have jointly asked every laboratory geneticist to be on call as a potential surveyor in their joint voluntary program.

[o]Laboratories using the CAP molecular pathology program must also participate in the relevant CAP/ACMG PT program.

its toll-free hotline (1-800-LAB-5678), and a CAP-published list of accredited laboratories.[P] As CAP is not deemed to accredit in areas of genetics, it does not make the results of its assessments of genetic test performance public.

The Task Force recommends that CAP/ACMG periodically publish, and make available to the public, a list of laboratories performing genetic tests satisfactorily under its voluntary program. Other PT programs should also publish the names of laboratories performing satisfactorily if they do not already do so. Until then, publication of results in voluntary proficiency and other quality assurance programs enable providers and consumers to select approved laboratories and also serve as an incentive for laboratories to participate in the CAP/ACMG quality assessment program. The information on laboratories performing satisfactorily should be readily accessible to consumers and providers.

Publishing the names of laboratories performing satisfactorily would advise users that labs not appearing on the list have either not submitted to external review or have not performed adequately.

Some managed care organizations select laboratories on financial as well as performance criteria. "I often run into problems when I try to recommend laboratory work for patients who are referred to us by HMOs. Quite often the HMOs will not give us permission to process the samples here at our laboratory, nor will they allow us to send the samples out to genetics labs which are familiar to us. Instead, they insist on sending samples out for analysis at labs which are unknown to us. Delays are frequent, and the quality of analysis is questionable. For example, the lab which we use for CF [cystic fibrosis] carrier testing currently screens for 32 mutations. We have gotten no indication from the HMO regarding the detection rate of the labs which they send samples to. It is therefore very difficult to counsel patients regarding results."--Genetic counselor in letter to the Task Force, 1997.

A genetic counselor at another center told the Task Force that the managed care network to which a man at risk of Huntington disease belonged objected to the high price of testing for the disorder in the laboratory used by her genetic center. The counselor sent his specimen to a lab acceptable to the insurer but unknown to her. After many months and phone calls, the counselor finally received a report of a negative result. The interpretation was inadequate. In the meantime, the man developed symptoms and signs of Huntington disease. The clinical laboratory refused to pay for a confirmatory test.

Directories of laboratories providing genetic tests (e.g.. HELIX--see chapter 5) should also publish information on listed laboratories' satisfactory participation in PT and other quality control programs specific for genetic tests. The Association for Molecular Pathology publishes information on the quality of laboratories, and the National Organization for Rare Diseases and the Alliance of Genetic

---

[P]R.C. Zastrow, President, College of American Pathologists, Communication, March 13, 1997, p. 7. The publication, "CAP Accredited Laboratories," can be ordered by calling 1-800-323-4040 (ext. 7531), or by writing to CAP Publications Order Department, 3235 Waukegan Road, Northfield IL, 60093. The fee for the publication is $20.

Support Groups make it publicly available. **Managed care organizations and other third-party payers should limit reimbursement for genetic tests to the laboratories on published lists of those satisfactorily performing genetic tests.** Implementation of this recommendation is especially important as more managed care organizations move to restrict access to laboratory services for their members to a single laboratory with whom each organization contracts. Such a laboratory might not have participated or performed satisfactorily in a quality control program.

A CENTRAL REPOSITORY OF CELL LINES AND DNA

Making cell lines or DNA containing disease-related mutations available to many laboratories would be useful in the validation of new tests, calibration, standardization, and quality control. To accomplish this, **appropriate specimens from patients, carriers, and controls should be available through a centralized repository in order to facilitate their availability to aid in analytical validation, improving quality, and other needs.** Resources such as the National Institute of General Medical Sciences' Human Genetic Mutant Cell Repository (housed at the Coriell Institute for Medical Research) and the American Type Culture Collection should be utilized. It should be impossible to trace samples in a repository to the individuals from whom they were obtained. The samples should not be used for any purpose from which a profit could be derived, such as the sale of unusual probes. A central repository of analytes for standardizing biochemical and other types of tests, including those used for screening, is also needed. Some mechanism for ensuring the composition and concentration of these standards, such as FDA review, is needed.

THE IMPORTANCE OF THE PRE- AND POST-ANALYTIC PHASES OF TESTING

In the pre-analytic phase, laboratories sometimes give information about the test to providers and consumers. Informed consent can be obtained, and data are requested from those to be tested. In the post-analytic phase, test results are given to the provider and patient, often with an interpretation. Genetic counseling services can be provided or arranged by laboratories, but are the responsibility of the referring provider.

Pre-analytic Phase

The Task Force is concerned about the quality of information made available to providers and consumers who are considering testing. Some materials have serious omissions that impair the ability of providers and consumers to make informed decisions about testing. In a comparison of four different brochures made available by organizations offering testing for genetic susceptibility to breast cancer, the Task Force found striking discrepancies. Physicians or consumers reading one brochure might, as a result, make a different decision than if they read another organization's brochure. It is the responsibility of health care providers, not the clinical laboratory, to provide information to the individual offered or considering testing, but material made available by laboratories is often used.

The completeness and accuracy of this material is, therefore, extremely important.

Obtaining informed consent helps ensure that the person voluntarily agrees to testing and has some understanding of the reasons for testing. Informed consent is appropriate for predictive genetic tests, particularly those for which stringent scrutiny is needed. **The Task Force is of the opinion**

Information in brochures on genetic testing. Of 115 pamphlets on genetic tests for providers and/or consumers collected from commercial and university-based genetic testing laboratories, fewer than half included statements about the accuracy of the test. These statements were often misleading. Some claimed the test was "over 99% accurate," but most of these did not specify whether the statements referred to analytic validity or to clinical sensitivity, specificity, or predictive value. Few of the pamphlets discussed risks of the test or even the intended purpose (see appendix 4).

Differences in information provided about genetic testing for breast cancer susceptibility. In late 1996, informational material was made available to the Task Force by four laboratories offering testing for inherited susceptibility mutations in the BRCA1 and BRCA2 genes. They differed markedly in content. One said that "population screening should be offered where feasible," but a second said [we must continue to collect data] "so that one day we will be able to offer appropriate screening guidelines based on firm clinical data..." This laboratory gave a risk of 59% for developing breast cancer by age 59 while a third gave a risk of 77% for developing breast cancer by age 59. The third lab said "Early [breast] cancer detection provides the best opportunity for reducing mortality from cancer" [presumably in those who are found to have inherited susceptibility mutations for breast cancer]. The brochure of a fourth laboratory said, "There is no surveillance or prevention strategy which is proven to decrease the mortality associated with carrying a [BRCA] mutation." The third lab said "prophylactic mastectomy does not completely eliminate the risk of breast cancer...However, the procedure substantially reduces the risk of breast cancer." The second lab said, "...there is very little data available as to how effective prophylactic surgery is at reducing breast cancer risk."

---

that laboratories should obtain documentation of informed consent when appropriate and should not perform an analysis if documentation is lacking. The most rigorous documentation is for the laboratory to be sent a signed copy of the patient's consent. It is less rigorous to ask the ordering physician to check a box on the laboratory requisition indicating that consent has been obtained.

Because of the complexities of assessment and interpretation, requisitions for many genetic tests require more intake information than those for virtually any other clinical laboratory procedure. In addition to routine information, genetic test requests often must include the reason for requesting the test, any relevant clinical or laboratory information, the person's age and ethnicity, and notation of family history of the disorder in question (along with a full pedigree for tests involving linkage analysis). If information that is critical to the performance or the interpretation of the test cannot be obtained, or if the information that is provided suggests that the patient is not an appropriate candidate for testing, the physician must be contacted. There is consensus, for instance, that minor children should not be tested for adult-onset disease for which no diagnostic or therapeutic interventions are needed before adulthood (see chapter 1). Yet some laboratories report testing children (see chapter 4 and appendix 3). Most authorities agree that healthy women without a family history of breast cancer should not be tested for inherited susceptibility mutations for breast cancer except under investigative protocols to gather data on the penetrance of these mutations, and that women with a family history of the disease should only be tested if an inherited susceptibility mutation is found in an affected relative.[5-7] Consequently, laboratories must ascertain the presence of a family history before accepting a specimen. At least one laboratory is offering testing to Ashkenazi Jewish women without a family history.[8] In general, laboratory personnel must be competent to recognize what information is needed and what the criteria are for accepting specimens. When in doubt, they must communicate with the ordering provider.

Post-analytic Phase

Increasingly, genetic tests will be requested by providers without much or any training in genetics. (Recommendations on ensuring provider competence appear in chapter 4.) Accurate and comprehensible interpretation of genetic test results by the clinical laboratories is critical to ensure that the provider understands the implications and can explain them to the persons who were tested. **Genetic test results must be written by the laboratory in a form that is understandable to the non-geneticist health care provider.** The quality of laboratories' written interpretations of genetic test results should be included in the overall assessment of laboratories providing genetic tests.

Some laboratories also make genetic counselors available to discuss results with physicians. If testing of other relatives is an option, a potential conflict of interest arises as the counselor might want to promote additional business.

Ensuring the Quality of Pre- and Post-analytic Phases

One way of improving laboratory performance is to have more rigorous standards with which laboratories must comply. The Task Force is of the opinion that not enough emphasis is placed on the pre- and post-analytic phases in CAP's molecular pathology and special chemistry programs. **The Task Force recommends that CAP and ACMG seek advice and input from consumer groups such as the Alliance of Genetic Support Groups, as well as from the National Society of Genetic Counselors (NSGC), on educational, psychological, and counseling issues in pre- and post-analytic components of genetic testing that are of direct concern to consumers.**

Under CLIA, the rating system used to establish the complexity of tests does not give sufficient weight to these phases (see box entitled Complexity Determinations under CLIA). CDC should consider how the pre- and post-analytic phases of predictive genetic testing can be given greater weight in CLIA standards and regulations.

DIRECT MARKETING OF GENETIC TESTS TO THE PUBLIC

Many clinical laboratories advertise the availability of tests directly to the public (see appendix 4). **Great care must be taken that information on genetic tests presented directly to the public is accurate and includes risks and limitations, as well as benefits.** The informational material should be sensitive to the knowledge level of the general public. In addition to describing the benefits and risks of the genetic test(s), including discrimination issues and the potential emotional impact on individuals and family members, the material should describe those for whom testing is appropriate (e.g., couples planning to have children for carrier tests, and individuals with a family history of a late-onset disorder for which genetic predispositions can be detected), and should emphasize that all genetic testing is voluntary, often requiring informed consent. **Consumers should discuss testing options with a health care provider competent in genetics prior to having specimens collected for analysis.**

The Task Force is concerned that no mechanism exists for the review of the accuracy of informational material on genetic tests made available either to providers or consumers, except for the labeling materials on kits that must be reviewed by FDA in premarket applications. As already noted, most genetic tests are marketed as services, not kits. Although complaints concerning inaccurate information can be made to FDA, the Federal Trade Commission, the Consumer Product Safety Commission, or the consumer protection divisions in the offices of most States' Attorneys General, harm could be done from exaggerated claims before complaints are filed or acted on. The external review of tests before they enter clinical use (see chapter 2) should include examination of proposed informational material.

In accord with laws in most States, clinical laboratories in the U.S. require that specimens for the vast majority of tests come from a physician or are reported to a physician. A few laboratories accept specimens for predictive genetic testing directly from consumers without the intervention of their own physician. In such cases, a physician affiliated with the testing laboratory, who is a specialist but may be previously unknown to the patient, can order the test. As DNA can be isolated and amplified from cells in saliva or scraped from the buccal mucosa, it is possible for lay people to collect their own specimens. FDA has the authority to regulate this practice if the laboratory supplies or requires use of a specially designated collection device or container to send specimens from the person's home to the laboratory. **The Task Force discourages advertising or marketing of predictive genetic tests to the public.**

INTERNATIONAL HARMONIZATION

At present, no mechanism exists to create international standards of laboratory quality and proficiency for genetic tests. Current United States regulations require any foreign laboratories performing clinical laboratory tests on U.S. residents to hold a CLIA certificate even if their nation's laboratory standards are more stringent than those of CLIA. **The Task Force recommends that efforts should be made to harmonize international laboratory standards to ensure the highest possible laboratory quality for genetic tests.** A proposed European Union Directive on "In Vitro Diagnostic Medical Devices," with which FDA is cooperating, will harmonize the situation for assessing medical devices including genetic test kits and reagents. This Directive, however, does not extend to tests provided as services, similar to the situation in the U.S.

REFERENCES

1. Kaback M, Lim-Steele J, Dabholkar D, Brown D, Levy N, Zeiger K: Tay-Sachs disease--carrier screening, prenatal diagnosis, and the molecular era. An international perspective, 1970 to 1993. The International TSD Data Collection Network. *JAMA* 1993;207:2307-2315.

2. Public Law 100-578: Clinical Laboratory Improvement Amendments of 1988. 1988;42 USC 263a.

3. Bogdanich W: False negative. Medical labs, trusted as largely error-free, are far from infallible. *Wall Street Journal* Feb. 2,1987:1.

4. Palomaki GE, Knight GJ, McCarthy JE, Haddow JE, Donhowe JM: Maternal serum screening for Down syndrome in the United States: A 1995 survey. *American Journal of Obstetrics and Gynecology* 1997;176:1046-1051.

5. Burke W, Kahn MJE, Garber JE, Collins FS: "First Do No Harm" applies to cancer susceptibility testing too. *Cancer Journal from Scientific American* 1996;2:250-252.

6. Weber B: Breast cancer susceptibility genes: Current challenges and future promises. *Annals of Internal Medicine* 1996;124:1088-1090.

7. Blue Cross and Blue Shield Association Technology Evaluation Center (TEC): Executive Summary of TEC Assessment on Genetic Testing for inherited BRCA1 or BRCA2 mutations. 1997.

8. Schulman JD, Stern HJ: Genetic predisposition testing for breast cancer. *Cancer Journal from Scientific American* 1997;2:244-249.

CHAPTER 4. IMPROVING PROVIDERS' UNDERSTANDINGS OF GENETIC TESTING

The increase in the number of disease-related genes that scientists have identified in recent years, particularly those in which inherited mutations increase susceptibility to common disorders, has engendered expectations that health care will be improved. The rate of increase of health care professionals trained and board-certified in medical genetics or genetic counseling has not kept pace

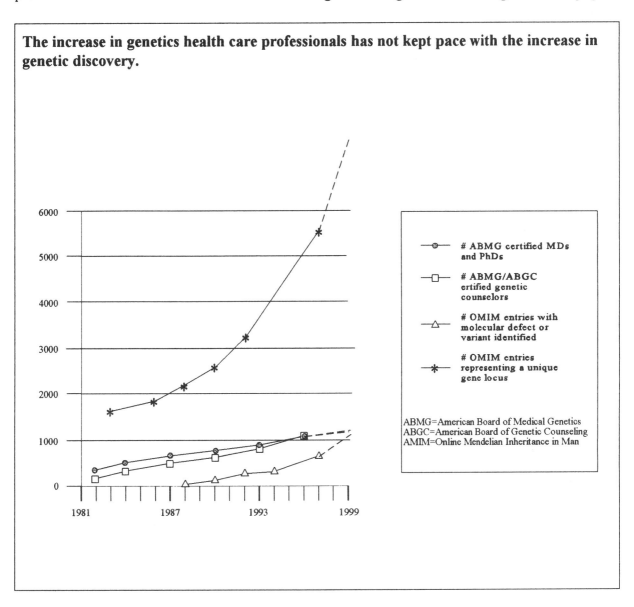

The increase in genetics health care professionals has not kept pace with the increase in genetic discovery.

with the rate of increase of genetic discovery and of potential demand for genetic tests. Although genetic professionals currently in practice or in training could meet a small increase in demand for genetic testing and counseling, their supply is insufficient to cope with even a doubling of the demand. Some commentators maintain that population carrier screening for just one condition, cystic fibrosis, would swamp the system.[1] Thus, if the demand for genetic testing increases, and the supply of genetics providers does not keep pace, other health care professionals will have to play a role, or new models of testing will have to be devised if the demands are to be met. In this chapter, we first delineate a role for non-genetic health care professionals in eliciting genetic risks and providing genetic tests. We then turn to the obstacles of having non-geneticists provide these services. We next consider policies for overcoming the obstacles and, finally, other models for providing genetic services.

A ROLE FOR NON-GENETIC HEALTH CARE PROFESSIONALS

In addition to the paucity of genetic specialists relative to the potential demand for genetic testing, there are other reasons why other professionals should be involved in genetic testing. First, few people have sufficient understanding of genetics to recognize whether or not they or their children are at increased risk of inherited disease. Therefore, health care professionals who provide care to most people have a responsibility to determine whether a high-risk situation is present. With the rise in managed care in the United States, these professionals are increasingly primary care providers who provide first-contact and continuing care and who may serve as gatekeepers for access to other specialists. Nevertheless, in the United States, many people can bypass primary care providers and seek care directly from specialists. Even when aware that a problem that concerns them might have a genetic origin, they are more likely to seek the care of the specialist who manages the problem when it becomes overt than the care of a geneticist. For instance, people concerned about an inherited susceptibility to cancer will go to an oncologist or surgeon more often than to a geneticist, and pregnant women concerned about birth defects or inherited disorders will ask their obstetrician instead of a geneticist. Consequently, non-genetic specialists, as well as primary care providers, become the gateway to genetic testing.

> **Growing importance of primary care.** "Primary care providers, who in the past referred their patients with genetic conditions to genetic specialists, are now more often the first to give their patients basic genetics information, determine their need for genetic services and decide where to secure such services. There is a growing awareness among medical professionals and consumers that new genetic technology is developing faster than the ability of these non-genetics medical professionals to fully consider the diagnostic, treatment and psychosocial implications of genetic tests and keep abreast of new clinical interventions." -- Alliance of Genetic Support Groups. *Partnership for Genetic Services Pilot Program.*

Second, primary care and other providers that people visit periodically are in an excellent position to elicit risk information. One important source of information about genetic risks is family history. When people receive their care from one source over a period of years, as is the ideal primary care situation, the provider is more likely to learn about family history as relatives become ill (whether they are in the provider's care or not) and, possibly, about other situations that raise the risks of genetic disease. If the source remains constant but the providers change, a single medical record used by all of the patient's providers gives the current provider an opportunity to recognize

60

risk factors, if the record is adequate. This advantage is lost when people change their source of care (at least until a universal medical record that people keep with them, such as a "smart card", is developed). Each new provider, including specialists, must attempt to ferret risk factors, including family history, again. The few studies that have been done show that family history, as elicited directly from people, does not always accurately reflect what medical records of relatives contain.[2-4] Despite their skill and expertise, genetic specialists who see a person only once, as is often the case in prenatal care, might not be able to elicit as complete a picture of risk factors for genetic disease as the primary care provider who sees the person repeatedly. Moreover, without recognition of genetic risk factors by primary care providers or other non-genetic health care providers, many people will never get to a genetic specialist.

Eliciting Risks of Genetic Disease in Healthy People

Family History. Although family history is an important source of information about risks of future genetic disease, it has limitations. We have already mentioned the problem of reliability. More importantly, its yield will depend on the mode of inheritance of the diseases of concern. It is most useful when diseases are inherited in a dominant or X-linked fashion. Some diseases inherited in these ways will, however, arise by new mutation and the family history will be negative. Eliciting a history of frequently-recurring common diseases that do not follow Mendelian inheritance might indicate the presence of inherited susceptibility, such as those for breast and colon cancer, or of polymorphisms that have been associated with disease. The family history is less likely to be informative for autosomal recessive diseases in which each parent of an affected child is an asymptomatic carrier. Eliciting a history of consanguinity in the parents points to an increased risk of autosomal recessive diseases in their children; the parents might each have inherited the same disease-related alleles from a common ancestor. This also explains why some autosomal diseases are higher in certain ethnic groups in the absence of consanguinity. Thus eliciting a person's ethnicity also becomes important. When people have many children, it is more likely that the family history will be positive for a recessive disease; on average, one out of four children will be affected. Adoption, the use of artificial insemination by donor sperm and multiple sexual partners, as well as people's greater mobility (removing them from the nuclear family), increase the difficulty in eliciting an informative family history. One systematic method of collecting family history data, and also establishing whether consanguinity is present, is the construction of a pedigree.

Past History. In view of the limitation of family history and ethnic origin, the health care provider must look for other ways of determining genetic risk factors for future disease. Some risk factors can also be elicited by interview. These include (1) the age of a pregnant woman; as maternal age increases, particularly over 35 years, the risk of Down syndrome and other chromosomal abnormalities in her fetus increases, and (2) past or present exposure to an environment that is more likely to result in disease in those with genetic predispositions, such as intake of fava beans or anti-malarial drugs in people with glucose-6-phosphate dehydrogenase deficiency, which has a higher frequency in people of African, Asian, and Mediterranean origin.

Genetic Testing. Finally, genetic testing can be used to elicit risks of future genetic disease. If the person's history is unrevealing and if the disease is a serious one that can be avoided by reproductive options, prevented, or more effectively treated by intervention in its presymptomatic stages than after symptoms appear, then population-wide screening can reduce the burden of the disease if it is utilized by many in the population. In the absence of an affected family member, carriers for autosomal recessive disease can be detected by genetic screening. Genetic testing can also confirm the presence of specific disease-related alleles in people with positive histories, pointing the way to specific interventions. Testing and screening should only be undertaken in clinical practice when the conditions for testing described in chapter 2 have been satisfied.

The question can be asked, why not simply screen everyone for disease-related alleles and bypass the family and past history? First, relatively few predictive tests applied on a population basis meet the criteria of validity and utility described in chapter 2. Second, even if they did, it would be extremely costly to test everyone. As the cost of the technology is reduced, this reason becomes less important. Third, the process of offering predictive genetic screening takes time. In accord with the principles of autonomy presented in chapter 1, people must be informed of the benefits and risks of screening and given an opportunity to decline it. Although this might be accomplished simply by brochures and other audio-visual aids, the effectiveness of these methods has not yet been established. Unless and until they are, providers will have to spend time explaining screening to potential users. Fourth, when the results come back, they have to be interpreted. As discussed in chapter 2, many genetic tests are not perfect predictors. The probability that disease will occur when the test result is negative, or that disease will not occur when the result is positive, both of which will be greater when populations rather than at-risk individuals are tested, must be explained.

The Role of Non-genetic Health Care Providers

With proper training and adequate knowledge of test validity, disease and mutation frequencies in the ethnic groups to whom they provide care, primary care providers and other non-genetic specialists can and should be the ones to offer predictive genetic tests to at-risk individuals. In some circumstances, for instance, when the family history is complicated or the symptomatology in relatives does not point to a clear diagnosis, referral to a genetic specialist is appropriate before offering testing. Unless there are other means of providing screening, such as through hospitals (for newborn screening) or public health facilities (see section on Other Models later in this chapter), non-genetic providers will almost always be involved in offering genetic screening, as well as testing. The role of non-genetic providers in interpreting test results is complex. The interpretation of positive results will often depend on further elicitation of risks, including family history. The options available to reduce risks will also have to be considered. Positive results can have implications for future children. Often they will also be of importance to other relatives with whom the person tested should be encouraged to communicate. For tests with imperfect sensitivity and those for susceptibility to common disorders, negative results do not eliminate the chance of future disease. A test's sensitivity and predictive value can also vary by ethnic group (e.g., the sensitivity of current CF carrier tests is much higher in Caucasians than in African or Asian Americans). Providers must be aware of these and other considerations in interpreting test results, and be capable of communicating risk information and its implications to those who are tested or their parents or guardians. Consultation with geneticists and/or genetic counselors might be appropriate.

OBSTACLES TO THE INVOLVEMENT OF NON-GENETIC PROFESSIONALS

Despite the advantages of non-genetic providers being the gateway to genetic testing, there are drawbacks. One is the limited knowledge of genetics and genetic tests of some non-geneticist providers. In a 1991 survey of physicians selected at random from ten states, non-genetic, non-academic physicians in five specialties (family practice, internal medicine, obstetrics-gynecology,

---

Providers' knowledge of a genetic test. The use and interpretation of a test for the adenomatous polyposis coli (APC) gene, which greatly increases the risk of one form of colon cancer, has been studied recently. One hundred and seventy-seven physicians ordered the test from a commercial laboratory. Over 80% of the physicians were non-geneticists. Eighty-eight of the people on whom the test was ordered were asymptomatic for colon cancer. The authors found that in 17% of all tests ordered, the indication for the test was not valid, that only 18.6 % of the patients received formal genetic counseling beforehand, and that only 16.9% (on whom this information was available) gave written-informed consent. In 31.6% of the tests, the physician's interpretation of the test result would have led to the misinforming of the patient. Often physicians did not know that a negative result did not alter the risk of colon cancer if no affected relative had an identifiable inherited mutation.[5]

One example of inappropriate use of the test for APC mutations was reported to the Task Force by a genetic counselor: "A pediatrician at an HMO ordered APC testing on a 5-year-old boy and 6-year-old girl. Testing was performed and the family was sent to our clinic for counseling. The gastroenterologist/oncologist and I were a bit uncomfortable with testing children so young because screening does not begin until age 10 for this condition and it is unclear how useful this information may be for the medical management of a 5- and 6-year-old. I believe it is the responsibility of the laboratory to at least educate those ordering tests like this about the generally accepted practices of not ordering presymptomatic testing on children unless there are current medical management issues."

---

pediatrics, and psychiatry) were able to correctly answer an average of 73.1% of questions deemed important by a panel of non-genetic providers who helped develop the questionnaire. Physicians who graduated from medical school between 1971 and 1985 scored significantly higher than those who graduated between 1950 and 1970. Having a genetics course in medical school was significantly associated with higher scores but was not as important a predictor as the year of graduation. Physicians in specialties that had been exposed to genetic problems in their practices (family physicians who delivered babies, pediatricians, and obstetrician-gynecologists) had significantly higher scores than physicians in the other specialties. Over one-third of family physicians who did not deliver babies, internists, and psychiatrists had scores of 65% correct or lower.[6]

In a 1996 survey on testing for genetic susceptibility to cancer, Burke and Press found that of the first 124 primary care physicians to respond, over 20% had not heard of a test for a genetic predisposition to breast cancer. (N. Press, personal communication)

Another drawback is the tendency of non-geneticist providers to be directive in situations in which reproductive options to avoid the conception or birth of an infant with a serious disorder are considered.[7-11] Primary care providers occasionally report that they will not offer a prenatal test to a patient who they are confident would not be interested in testing.[8] Whether the provider, even one with a continuing relationship with the patient, really does know the patient's attitudes on this subject and, if so, is justified in withholding information, is debatable. Recently, it has been recognized that nondirectiveness might not be achievable and might not be something that patients always want.[12-15] Nevertheless, because of past efforts to deny people the opportunity to reproduce because they possessed presumably heritable traits,[16,17] and the need to respect personal autonomy in reproductive matters, efforts to steer people toward a particular reproductive decision are undesirable (see chapter 1).

When safe, effective, and widely acceptable interventions are available for people with positive predictive test results, the role of nondirectiveness is much less of an issue. When interventions are not of proven safety and effectiveness, people should be told that is the case and should decide for themselves whether they want testing and, if they do and subsequently have a positive test result, whether they want the unproven intervention.

It is not clear that primary care providers could devote the time that informing patients about risks and benefits of genetic tests often entails. The average time spent counseling new patients in genetics or prenatal clinics exceeds 1 hour.[18] The median time of counseling for molecular genetic testing is 1 hour, not counting preparation (record review) or clerical and administrative time.[19]

POLICIES FOR IMPROVING THE ABILITY OF NON-GENETIC HEALTH CARE PROFESSIONALS TO BE INVOLVED IN GENETIC TESTING

The Task Force considered a number of strategies, both long and short-term, for improving the ability of non-genetic health care professionals to provide genetic services safely and effectively.

Greater Public Knowledge of Genetics
A knowledge base on genetics and genetic testing should be developed for the general public. Without a sound knowledge base, informed decisions are impossible and claims of autonomy and informed consent suspect. People who are more knowledgeable will grasp more readily the issues raised by providers when they offer tests. This could diminish the time needed for education and counseling without reducing consideration of the implications of testing. Policies for improving public understanding of genetics and genetic tests are beyond the scope of the Task Force. A number of private and public organizations have, through public statement and program investment, strongly endorsed the need for large-scale educational programs.[a] Educating the public in genetics presents

---

[a] Public education demonstration projects have received support from the NIH and DOE Ethical, Legal, and Social Implications program and from the Genetic Services Branch of the Maternal and Child Health Bureau. The Branch has sponsored educational projects, including curriculum development and classroom models adaptable for national dissemination. The Human Genome Education Model Project of Georgetown University and the Alliance of Genetic Support Groups (supported by NIH) are working with the leadership of seven

enormous challenges. Many people's views of how traits are inherited are inconsistent with Mendelian inheritance.[20] **New models of providing education and counseling to patients and other consumers are needed.**

Ethnic groups differ in their perceptions of disease origins and what should be done to avert disease.[21-23] Moreover, identifying a genetic variant that has a much higher frequency in some ethnic groups than in others could have a stigmatizing effect on that group. In keeping with the overarching principles described in chapter 1, sensitivity to cultural differences is of paramount importance. Unfortunately, minorities are seriously under-represented in the field of genetics.

Professional Education

Undergraduate and Graduate Medical Education. **The Task Force encourages the development of genetics curricula in medical school and residency training to enable all physicians to recognize inherited risk factors in patients and families, and appreciate issues in genetic testing and the use of genetic services.** A committee of the American Society of Human Genetics has published a list of objectives for medical school courses and the skills and attitudes they should engender in medical students.[24]

According to a 1995 survey by the Association of American Medical Colleges (AAMC), 68 of 125 four-year medical schools in the U.S. required genetics courses in their curricula (personal communication from Al Salas, Association of American Medical Colleges to Task Force, July 16, 1997). Although genetics is sometimes an integral part of other basic science courses in some other medical schools, the Task Force is concerned that genetics is not being taught adequately to all medical students. The AAMC survey also found that most genetics is taught in the first 2 (basic science) years of medical school. Consequently, many clinical aspects will not receive adequate attention. The Task Force is not suggesting that the courses be moved to the clinical years but that clinical departments pay greater attention to genetic issues.

As provider-patient communication is critical in offering genetic tests and counseling about them, consumers should be involved in the planning and implementation of new curricula in genetics. The Partnership for Genetic Services Pilot Program, just launched by the Alliance of Genetic Support Groups, and supported by public and private funds, has, as its goal, improving medical student and provider understanding, sensitivity, and competence in delivering genetic services. It will do this by exposing medical students and physicians-in-training to relevant community resource systems and illustrative presentations by consumers. Partnerships between consumers and clinical genetics providers, primary care practitioners, medical school faculty, and managed care administrators have been established.

---

national allied health organizations to develop educational materials and enhance understanding about genetics and associated ethical, legal, and social issues.

<u>Licensure and Certification</u>. **The likelihood that genetics will be covered in curricula will improve if relevant genetics questions are included in general licensure and specialty board certification examinations, and if correctly answering a proportion of the genetics questions is needed to attain a passing score.** Medical school curriculum and residency review committees, which exist at both the local medical school and hospital levels and at the national level, define teaching content based on core material needed for clinical practice, recent advances, and questions on board examinations. Those who prepare board examinations, the National Board of Medical Examiners for medical students, and the various specialty boards for specialty certification, derive questions from material they think important, yet questions involving genetics are sparse and sometimes inappropriate. The American Council of Graduate and Medical Education (ACGME), is the umbrella organization for boards and residency review committees, and also contributes importantly to residency training content. The Task Force encourages ACGME, as well as residency review committees, to consider the importance of graduate training in genetics. The Task Force is pleased that the American Board of Obstetrics and Gynecology and the Society of Perinatal Obstetricians have acknowledged the importance of teaching genetics, including ethical aspects, by including questions on the basic obstetrics and gynecology exams, as well as on the subspecialty board exams of Maternal-Fetal Medicine.[b]

Traditionally, much medical school education and residency training occurred on the wards of hospitals. Those responsible for education and training have begun to recognize that most medical care is provided in ambulatory settings and that the delivery of care in those areas presents challenges for education. Genetic testing is a prime example. Moreover, teaching about genetic tests, including such issues as analytic and

> **Genetics questions on the U.S. Medical Licensing Examination (for medical students).** The examination was reviewed by a delegation from the Association of Professors of Human Medical Genetics and the American Society of Human Genetics. On the three parts of the examination, the delegation found that less than 5% of the questions required knowledge of genetics. Of these, only about one-third dealt with important genetic principles. More than two-thirds of all the genetic questions were on the first examination. Most of the few genetic items on either the second or third examinations tested specific facts related to individual genetic diseases rather than important principles of medical genetics. Several "correct answers" were considered wrong by the delegation because recent genetic discoveries were ignored. Family history and genetic diseases were sometimes used as extraneous information, giving the impression that they were trivial or unimportant.--Report on Review of the U.S. Medical Licensing Examination Test Materials in Medical Genetics. J.M. Friedman, M.D. Ph.D., Chair of the Genetics delegations visiting the National Board of Medical Examiners, December 4-5, 1995.

---

[b]R.C. Cefalo, President, American Board of Obstetrics and Gynecology, Communication to the Task Force, March 10, 1997; J.E. Ferguson, Board member, Society of Perinatal Obstetricians, E-mail communication to the Task Force, March 10, 1997.

clinical validity, introduces students and residents to general problems of reliability and test sensitivity and specificity, which are important for a much wider range of clinical laboratory tests.

In a rapidly changing field such as genetics, curricula that focus on current discoveries and do not lay a basic framework will rapidly become obsolete. The Task Force is particularly concerned that underlying concepts of genetics are not adequately learned by all physicians. Equally important are the means of communicating genetic concepts and risks to patients. Although the tests will change, many aspects of patient-provider communication will not, although here, too, much research is beginning to explore the nature of these interactions.

Continuing Medical Education. The full beneficial effects of improving medical school and residency curricula in genetics will not be felt for many years. Consequently, improving the ability of providers currently in practice to offer and interpret genetic tests correctly is of paramount importance. The Task Force vigorously debated the question of whether this goal could best be accomplished by a "carrot" or "stick" approach. An early position taken by the Task Force was: "Some documentation of continuing education in the area of human and medical genetics should be required for physicians offering genetic tests, including primary care providers."[25(p.24)] As the Task Force deliberated, it developed doubts as to whether continuing education could accomplish this goal and whether a requirement would

> **Task Force Goals of a Model Curriculum for Providers of Genetic Tests.** Providers should:
> - Be able to produce a reliable pedigree and assess risks of genetic disorders.
> - Recognize parameters of eligibility for each test.
> - Understand and be able to explain the risks and benefits associated with the test being considered.
> - Learn how to administer informed consent to patients being offered genetic tests.
> - Become familiar with genetic counseling strategies and principles as they relate to genetic tests.
> - Be able to explain the implications of the test to patients considering testing.
>
> --Subcommittee on Provider Education, Katherine Schneider, Chair

accomplish the Task Force's objective. The Task Force was also concerned that such a requirement would be difficult to enforce. The need to demonstrate competence is discussed further in the next section, but the point the Task Force wishes to emphasize is the need for each specialty to recognize that all of those who are certified in that specialty appreciate the importance of genetics and genetic tests relevant to that specialty. **In addition to basic curricula already considered, the Task Force recommends that each specialty involved with the care of patients with disorders with genetic components should design its own curriculum for continuing education in genetics.**

Administrators and other nonphysician personnel who triage patients and/or make coverage or reimbursement decisions, such as those in managed care organizations, should also have knowledge of the benefits and risks of genetic testing.

Demonstrating Provider Competence

Hospitals and managed care organizations, on advice from the relevant medical specialty departments, should request evidence of competence before permitting providers to order predictive genetic tests defined as needing stringent scrutiny or to counsel about them. Periodic,

Periodic, systematic medical record review, with feedback to providers, should also be used to ensure appropriate use of genetic tests.

Prerequisites. If hospitals and managed care organizations are to request evidence of competence, three prerequisites must be met. First, a mechanism must be in place for deciding which tests need evidence of competence. The Task Force believes that this should be one of the tasks of the proposed Secretary's Advisory Committee described in chapter 1. Second, competence must be defined. This can be accomplished by agreement between representatives of the non-genetic specialties involved in testing and of the genetics profession. Guidelines for establishing competence developed at the national level, e.g., by professional societies, which could be facilitated by the proposed Secretary's Advisory Committee, are ultimately preferable, but local agreements might be more readily reached when a test first becomes available. Third, easily accessible educational modules must be available to enable providers to gain competence. (We discuss some possibilities in the next section.) Unless continuing education opportunities are readily available, providers will be deterred from gaining sufficient knowledge of genetics to enable them to offer genetic tests appropriately to their patients.

Although little precedent exists for asking for a demonstration of competence before ordering tests that will be performed primarily in ambulatory settings, there are several reasons why some predictive genetic tests (those requiring stringent scrutiny) should be ordered only by those with demonstrated competence. Some of these reasons are important primarily to the person being tested, some to the provider offering the test, and some to those paying for the test.

- People need to have sufficient information about the clinical validity of the test to decide whether the test is appropriate for them. Providers must be able to give them the requisite information.
- The implications of a positive or negative test result might influence people's decision to be tested. Providers must be aware of the implications and discuss them with the people considering testing.
- People's autonomy must be respected especially when procedures for avoiding the conception or birth of a child with a genetic disease are options following a positive test result. Atonomy is also crucial when the interventions in those with positive test results have not been proven to be safe and effective. Providers must recognize these situations, understand the need to respect autonomy, and be able to communicate information in the least directive manner possible.
- The results of some predictive genetic tests will indicate that relatives might be at risk of genetic disease. Providers must be prepared to discuss why and how the person tested should communicate with relatives and what the relatives should do.
- Providers could face legal liability if they order a test inappropriately or if they communicate results to relatives (except in extreme circumstances--see chapter 1) or unrelated third parties without the consent of the person tested.
- Third parties paying for the test, including managed care organizations, will not want to reimburse if the test has been ordered unnecessarily or inappropriately.

Enforcement. The Task Force does not favor requiring organizations to establish competence requirements. It believes self-interest, as just discussed, will lead many organizations to set them. Nor is it necessary for laboratories to request documentation of competence before they will perform a genetic test. Providers who work for organizations who do credential for genetic testing would place themselves in legal jeopardy if they ordered the test without having the credential. Providers who do not work with an organization that credentials, for instance a solo practitioner in private practice, might be competent to order genetic tests but will have no credential to present. In their survey, Burke and Press found that one quarter of respondents disagreed strongly with a suggestion that physicians should be required to undergo a brief certification in genetics before they could order susceptibility tests; less than 19% agreed strongly. The majority expressed moderate support for this position. (N. Press, personal communication, June 1997) As discussed in chapter 3, the laboratory does have a responsibility to determine from the requisition that the test is indicated, and that, when appropriate, informed consent has been obtained from the person to be tested or his or her legal guardian.

Medical record audits assure managed care and other organizations that providers are satisfying standards of care. The feedback given to providers also serves as a valuable reenforcement to what has previously been learned. Audits of records for frequently-ordered medical tests should be considered. The Joint Commission on Accreditation of Healthcare Organizations (JCAHO) and

---

Criteria for assessing medical records for competence in genetic testing. Medical records should be audited for appropriate use of frequently-ordered predictive genetic tests. The criteria for demonstrating competence include, but are not limited to:

- Family history/pedigree present and adequate, with evidence of periodic updating.
- Appropriate indications for offering the test.
- Offering the test when it is indicated.
- Documentation of informed consent when appropriate.
- Appropriate description of the test result given to the patient, including the options for followup.

These criteria could be applied to fairly frequently-occurring situations, such as breast or colon cancer in which, to begin with, taking of a family history is documented.

---

the National Committee for Quality Assurance (NCQA) should consider asking hospitals and other health care organizations to develop continuous quality improvement programs focusing on genetic testing.

Assisting Providers in Gaining Competence in Genetics

When organizations begin to require that providers have demonstrable competence in genetics, the means of acquiring that competence must be available. The American College of Medical Genetics is working with other specialties to set guidelines and standards to assist in the development of curricula. It responded to a request from the American Society of Clinical Oncologists to assist it setting up "train the trainer" modules for oncologists who can then train others in their specialty. ACMG would be responsive to requests from other organizations as well.

The Task Force endorses the recent establishment of a National Coalition for Health Professional Education in Genetics (NCHPEG) by the American Medical Association, the American Nurses Association, and the National Human Genome Research Institute. The Coalition should work in consultation with non-genetic professional societies, such as the Association of American Medical Colleges, the American Council on Graduate and Medical Education, and genetic societies, such as the American College of Medical Genetics, the National Society of Genetic Counselors, the International Society of Nurses in Genetics, and appropriate consumer groups to encourage the development of core curricula in genetics. It should encourage input by consumers in the development of these curricula. In order to avoid duplication, the Coalition should serve as a registry and clearinghouse for, and disseminator of, information about various curricula and educational programs, grants, and training pilot programs in genetics education. It should encourage professional societies to track the effectiveness of their respective educational programs.

The Task Force welcomes the interest of the Agency for Health Care Policy and Research (AHCPR) in helping the Coalition develop a research agenda in health education.

In 1994, the Maternal and Child Health Bureau (MCHB) of the Health Resources and Services Administration, through its Genetic Services Branch, began soliciting grant applications to

---

The National Coalition for Health Professional Education in Genetics. The Coalition emerged in response to the growing need for the exchange of information and coordination of genetics education activities at a national level, and is comprised of leaders from approximately 100 diverse health care professional organizations, consumer and voluntary groups, government agencies, industry, managed care organizations, and genetics professional organizations. Goals of the Coalition are: to stimulate and formalize interest in establishing genetics education as a top priority for health care professional organizations and their memberships; to create mechanisms for collaboration between member organizations; to identify and coordinate existing and future genetics activities for health care professionals; and to develop new initiatives to meet identified needs. Top priorities are the development of a comprehensive, World Wide Web-based genetics information center; the development of a core curriculum in genetics for health professionals, to serve as a template that can be modified according to discipline; and the provision of incentives for providers to learn about genetics, such as incorporation of genetics questions into certification and licensure exams.

---

strengthen genetics in primary care. Thus far nine programs have been funded and several more are expected to be funded in 1998.[c] At least one educational module is available on the World Wide Web under MCH NetLink (http://www.ichp.edu/mchb/netlink/index.html). Others will appear shortly. Another

---

[c]The nine organizations receiving MCHB support thus far are: The Foundation for Blood Research, Scarborough ME; the Association of Asian Pacific Community Health Organizations, Oakland, CA; Laboratory of Medical Genetics, Birmingham AL; University of Texas Health Science Center at San Antonio, TX; Cornell University Medical College, New York, NY; Oregon Health Sciences University, Portland OR; Washington State Department of Health, Seattle WA; University of Washington, Seattle WA; University of Puerto Rico Medical Sciences Campus, San Juan, PR.

MCHB grantee, the Council of Regional Networks for Genetic Services (CORN) has recently issued its Guidelines for Clinical Genetic Services for the Public's Health.[26] MCHB has also asked CORN to prepare national guidelines that can be used for comprehensive followup care of children and families with rare metabolic disorders that can be used by purchasers and service providers in negotiating contracts with managed care plans.

CDC has developed a Public Health Training Network that can be adapted to provide information about genetics. The network often employs satellite broadcasting to multiple receiving sites with phone communication from the sites to permit two-way communication. The Network also develops material for Internet presentations and self-study, computer-based training modules. A wide range of subjects have been presented, including basic epidemiology, specific disease management, immunizations, and managing laboratories under CLIA. The format includes lectures, panel discussions, and videos.

A major problem in all educational endeavors is finding the "teachable moment," the time at which people, including health care providers, are receptive to new information and are most likely to retain it. These moments arise when providers are asked questions about genetic tests or when charts are flagged because the patient fulfills criteria for being offered a genetic test. Clearly, more people are asking providers questions about genetic tests. Computerized medical records or self-completing questionnaires (see box entitled Educational Module to Assist Physicians in Recognizing Genetic Risks) can generate flags to advise providers to offer genetic tests to people at risk. Printouts of background information, when flags are raised, could assist the provider. A 1-800 hotline that providers (and the public, perhaps,) can call to learn more about specific genetic tests, including availability and indications for their use, should be established by NCHPEG or some of its governmental and private constituent organizations.

> **Educational module to assist physicians in recognizing genetic risks.** Supported in part by the Maternal and Child Health Bureau, the Foundation for Blood Research in Scarborough Maine, has developed a series of materials for distribution to providers of prenatal care. The first is a short Genetic History Questionnaire to be completed by new obstetrical patients. The questions act as a screen for more than twenty common genetic conditions. When a "Yes" answer raises a flag for risk of one or more of these conditions, the provider can turn to the relevant section in the accompanying Office Guide, which contains a secondary questionnaire designed to help determine the person's or couple's level of risk. Each section also contains recommendations for followup, information on appropriate testing (including availability and typical cost), informational material for patients, local and national resources for information and support, general information about the disorder, frequently asked questions (with the answers), and references.

OTHER MODELS

Nursing

The overall time that physicians spend talking with patients on all subjects is usually less than the time that genetic counselors spend informing people about genetic tests and their implications.

The nursing profession has recognized that nurses have much to offer in helping people appreciate the benefits and risks of genetic testing.[27,28] Nurses can not only counsel (when trained) but also perform a wide range of activities in health care that genetic counselors are not qualified to do. Nurses are also in much greater supply. Nurses have been shown to be effective in providing education for testing for genetic susceptibility to cancer.[29] Oncology nurses increasingly view themselves as genetic health care professionals.[d] One nursing organization told the Task Force, "We see genetic education as core content in nursing education at both the undergraduate and advanced levels."[e] Nurses have played a large role in genetic counseling in the United Kingdom for many years.[30] A study currently under way in the U.S. is comparing the ability of nurse practitioners and genetic counselors in educating and counseling about testing for genetic susceptibility to breast cancer. (G. Geller, work in progress) Nurses should be provided with additional education and training that can increase their effectiveness in providing education for people undergoing genetic testing.

Community and Public Health

Although population-wide screening can be integrated into personal health care--prenatal screening in obstetrics provides a good example--different models have been used. In each case, screening has been undertaken because it permitted detection of many more at-risk subjects than would have been possible by using family histories. In this way, the opportunities for avoidance, prevention, or effective treatment are greater than waiting for symptoms to appear. For instance, diagnosing an older infant or child with phenylketonuria does little to prevent her retardation although it alerts the family to its risk of having additional children with that disease. Newborn screening, on the other hand, prevents retardation of the first child and all others who carry the disease-causing genotype (see appendix 5).

In many states, it is the responsibility of the hospital in which the baby is born to conduct screening. This model takes advantage of the fact that most babies are born in the hospital, making it easy to reach them. It is not advantageous once babies are discharged. Nevertheless, as testing for more inherited conditions become available and the safety and effectiveness of treating them neonatally is established, newborn screening could expand markedly.

Community-centered screening presents another model. Tay-Sachs carrier screening was originally organized at the community level; health care professionals who staffed the sites generally volunteered their time. The success of this effort depended on the cooperation of a cohesive community committed to screening. Nevertheless, not everyone in the ethnic group at risk came for screening and other methods had to be devised to reach them (see appendix 6). In the 1970s, and to a lesser extent today, sickle cell screening was performed at community sites and in health department clinics. For reasons discussed in appendix 6, this screening was not always a great success. Today, screening newborns for sickle cell anemia is part of many States' newborn screening programs.[31] Sickle cell screening is succeeding in lowering morbidity and mortality from this disease among

---

[d]K. Mooney, President, Oncology Nursing Society, Communication to Task Force, March 7, 1997.

[e]P.J.Reidy. President, Association of Women's Health, Obstetric and Neonatal Nurses, Communication to Task Force, March 10, 1997.

African-American children.[32] Any effort to initiate community-based genetic screening must have the active support of the community. Particularly when minority communities are involved, the program must be sensitive to issues of discrimination and provide sufficient resources for education and counseling.

Many other disorders are spread throughout diverse communities and it would be a Herculean task to organize community-based screening. Screening could be offered in health department clinics, mobile vans, or other sites, but not all segments of the population are likely to utilize them. A greater chance of breaching confidentiality is possible at community and health department sites than in the privacy of the traditional provider-patient relationship. Informed consent might not always be obtained.[33] Traditionally, health departments have been most involved in clinical care when there were well-accepted interventions (such as immunizations or tuberculosis control) without which the health of the public would be jeopardized. It might be difficult for public health personnel to appreciate that someone who refuses genetic screening is not jeopardizing the health of the public.

Before these new models can be investigated, additional training of the personnel involved is necessary. **Schools of nursing, public health, and social work need to strengthen their training programs in genetics.**[f]

---

[f]The Human Genome Education Model Project of Georgetown University and the Alliance of Genetic Support Groups are creating training programs in genetics for two national social work organizations.

REFERENCES

1. Wilfond BS, Fost N: The cystic fibrosis gene: Medical and societal implications for heterozygote detection. *JAMA* 1990;263:2777-2783.

2. Mendlewicz J, Fleiss JL, Cataldo M, Rainer JD: Accuracy of the family history method in affective illness. Comparison with direct interviews in family studies. *Archives of General Psychiatry* 1975;32:309-314.

3. Kee F, Tiret L, Robo JY, et al: Reliability of reported family history of myocardial infarction. *BMJ* 1993;307:1528-1530.

4. Offit K, Brown K: Quantitating familial cancer risk: A resource for clinical oncologists. *Journal of Clinical Oncology* 1994;12:1724-1736.

5. Giardiello FM, Brensinger JD, Petersen GM, et al: The use and interpretation of commercial APC gene testing for familial adenomatous polyposis. *New England Journal of Medicine* 1997;336:823-827.

6. Hofman KJ, Tambor ES, Chase GA, Geller G, Faden RR, Holtzman NA: Physicians' knowledge of genetics and genetic tests. *Academic Medicine* 1993;68:625-631.

7. Geller G, Tambor ES, Chase GA, Hofman KJ, Faden RR, Holtzman NA: Incorporation of genetics in primary care practice. Will physicians do the counseling and will they be directive? *Archives of Family Medicine* 1993;2:1119-1125.

8. Geller G, Holtzman NA: A qualitative assessment of primary care physicians' perceptions about the ethical and social implications of offering genetic testing. *Qualitative Health Research* 1995;5:97-116.

9. Holmes-Siedle MN, Rynanen M, Lindenbaum RH: Parental decisions regarding termination of pregnancy following prenatal detection of sex chromosome abnormality. *Prenatal Diagnosis* 1987;7:239-244.

10. Marteau TM, Plenicar M, Kidd J: Obstetricians presenting amniocentesis to pregnant women: Practice observed. *Journal of Reproductive and Infant Psychology* 1993;11:3-10.

11. Marteau TM, Drake H, Bobrow M: Counselling following diagnosis of a fetal abnormality: The differing approaches of obstetricians, clinical geneticists, and genetic nurses. *Journal of Medical Genetics* 1994;31:864-867.

12. Bernhardt BA: Empirical evidence that genetic counseling is directive: Where do we go from here? *American Journal of Human Genetics* 1997;60:17-20.

13. Michie S, Bron F, Bobrow M, Marteau TM: Nondirectiveness in genetic counseling: An empirical study. *American Journal of Human Genetics* 1997;60:40-47.

14. Kessler S: Psychological aspects of genetic counseling. VII. Thoughts on directiveness. *Journal of Genetic Counseling* 1992;1:9-17.

15. Clarke A: Is non-directive genetic counselling possible? *The Lancet* 1991;338:998-1001.

16. Kevles DJ: *In the name of eugenics.* New York, Alfred A. Knopf Inc. 1985.

17. Reilly P: *The surgical solution: A history of involuntary sterilization in the United States.* Baltimore, The Johns Hopkins University Press; 1991.

18. Bernhardt BA, Pyertiz RE: The economics of clinical genetics services. III. Cognitive genetics services are not self-supporting. *American Journal of Human Genetics* 1989;44:288-293.

19. Surh LC, Wright PG, Cappelli M, et al: Delivery of molecular genetic services within a health care system: Time analysis of the clinical workload. *American Journal of Human Genetics* 1995;56:760-768.

20. Richards M: Lay and professional knowledge of genetics and inheritance. *Public Understanding of Science* 1996;5:217-230.

21. Angel R, Thoits P: The impact of culture on the cognitive structure of illness. *Cultural Medical Psychiatry* 1987;11:465-494.

22. Punales-Morejon D, Penchaszadeh VB: Psychosocial aspects of genetic counseling: Cross-cultural issues. *Birth Defects* 1992;28:11-15.

23. Dibble SL, Vanoni JM, Miaskowski C: Women's attitudes toward breast cancer screening procedures: Differences by ethnicity. *Women's Health Issues* 1997;7:47-54.

24. American Society of Human Genetics Information and Education Committee: Report from the ASHG Information and Education Committee: Medical school core curriculum in genetics. *American Journal of Human Genetics* 1995;56:535-537.

25. Task Force on Genetic Testing: Interim principles. *Available at www.med.jhu.edu/tfgtelsi* 1996.

26. Council of Regional Networks for Genetic Services (CORN): Guidelines for Clinical Genetic Services for the Public's Health. 1997;First Edition, CORN, Atlanta GA.

27. Monsen RB: Nursing takes leading role in genetics education: Coalition formed to increase provider awareness on genetics technologies. *American Nurse* 1996;28:11

28. Anderson GW: The evolution and status of genetics education in nursing in the United States 1983-1995. *Image The Journal of Nursing Scholarship* 1996;28:101-106.

29. Lerman C, Biesecker B, Benkendorf JL, et al: Controlled trial of pretest education approaches to enhance infomed decision-making for BRCA1. *Journal of the National Cancer Institute* 1997;89:148-157.

30. Williams A: Genetic counseling. A nurse's perspective. In Clarke A (ed): *Genetic Counseling. Practice and Principles.* New York, Routledge; 1994:44-62.

31. Hiller EH, Landenburger G, Natowicz MR: Public participation in medical policy making and the status of consumer autonomy: The example of newborn screening programs in the United States. *American Journal of Public Health* 1997;87:1280-1288.

32. Vichinsky E, Hurst D, Earles A, Kleman K, Lubin B: Newborn screening for sickle cell disease: Effect on mortality. *Pediatrics* 1988;81:749-755.

33. Farfel MR, Holtzman NA: Education, consent, and counseling in sickle cell screening programs: Report of a survey. *American Journal of Public Health* 1984;74:373-375.

CHAPTER 5. GENETIC TESTING FOR RARE INHERITED DISORDERS

The vast majority of single-gene (Mendelian) disorders are rare, occurring less often than 1 in 10,000 live births. Exceptions are sickle cell anemia, cystic fibrosis, thalassemia, and Tay-Sachs disease in some populations, and heterozygous familial hypercholesterolemia, Duchenne muscular dystrophy, and the hemophilias more generally. Phenylketonuria, for which newborns are routinely screened, occurs in slightly less than 1 in 10,000 births. Most of the several thousand other known inherited diseases occur much less frequently, but their *combined* incidence is by no means rare. Between 10 and 20 million Americans may suffer from one of the several thousand known rare diseases over their lifetimes.[1(p. xiii)] With the discovery of the role of inherited mutations in common diseases, such as breast and colon cancer and Alzheimer disease (albeit in a small proportion of affected people), the Task Force is concerned that research might shift away from the multitude of rare diseases. Commercial genetic test developers, for instance, expend a greater effort on the common, complex disorders than on rare ones (see table 3, appendix 3). **The development and maintenance of tests for rare genetic diseases must continue to be encouraged.**

Congress recognized the need to provide incentives for the development of drugs for rare diseases when it passed the Orphan Drug Act in 1983.[2] To stimulate research and development, it granted a 7-year period of market exclusivity for unpatented drugs, a tax credit to offset the cost of drug development (the tax credit expired in 1994), and government grants and contracts to help defray costs of clinical studies. Over 300 grants have been awarded, primarily to support the development of drugs and biologics. (Personal communication, Dr. John V. Kelsey, Office of Orphan Products Development, FDA, February 22, 1996) In 1988, Congress added medical devices, authorizing government grants and contracts for "defraying the costs of developing medical devices for rare diseases or conditions."[3] Devices now account for about 10% of all orphan products receiving assistance under the Act.

As part of the Safe Medical Devices Act of 1990, Congress enacted the Humanitarian Device Exemption "to encourage the discovery and use of devices intended to benefit patients in the treatment and diagnosis of diseases or conditions that affect fewer than 4,000 individuals in the United States."[4] The incentive to device manufacturers is temporary authorization to market the device without meeting the effectiveness requirements of FDA. The exemption lasts for 18 months, although it can be renewed for up to 5 years. During the period of the exemption, the manufacturer cannot obtain a profit on device sales; the device must receive pre-market approval before a profit mark-up can be included in the price. In addition to the special incentives under these Acts, approximately 20% of the National Institutes of Health (NIH) budget funds research that is related to rare diseases, of which about 90-95% are inherited. (Personal communication, Steven Groft, Director Office of Rare Diseases, NIH, October-November 1996)

There is no uniform definition of a rare disease. The Orphan Drug Act (ODA) defines orphan disease as one affecting less than 200,000 persons in the U.S., or approximately 1 in 1,250 Americans. For devices (which include genetic tests), the 1988 ODA Amendments define rare disease as "any disease or condition that occurs so infrequently in the United States that there is no reasonable expectation that a medical device...will be developed without [financial] assistance."[a] As already noted, the Humanitarian Device Exemption of the Safe Medical Devices Act of 1990 applies to diseases or conditions that affect fewer than 4,000 persons in the United States (1 in 62,500 Americans). It is silent on what constitutes a disease or condition (e.g., whether rare variants of a common genetic disease constitute a separate disease, or whether carriers are excluded). The carrier (heterozygote) frequency for autosomal recessive disorders with an incidence of 1 in 10,000 is 1 in 50.

Of great concern to the Task Force is the dissemination of information related to the diagnosis and management of rare diseases, the continuing availability of tests for their diagnosis and for predicting risk of future disease, and, finally, the quality of laboratories performing genetic tests for rare diseases. We consider these topics in turn in the remainder of this chapter.

DISSEMINATION OF INFORMATION ABOUT RARE DISEASES

Research Activity

The NIH Office of Rare Diseases (ORD), founded in 1994, maintains a database of clinical studies involving rare diseases that are funded by NIH. At the end of 1996, approximately 300 studies were contained in the database. ORD plans to expand the database to include clinical research supported by private organizations, including the biotechnology and pharmaceutical industries. When fully operational, the database will contain abstracts of studies, enrollment criteria, and the names of principal investigators and how to contact them. The database is available to patients, providers, and other researchers on the World Wide Web at http://rarediseases.info.nih.gov/pages. In the future, people may be able to contact principal investigators of clinical studies through the databases. ORD would also like to coordinate rare disease research by the establishment of an information center, which would also respond to inquiries about rare genetic disorders. Funds have been authorized but not appropriated.

The Metabolic Information Network (MIN) (Dallas, Texas) is a registry containing medical information on approximately 10,000 living and deceased patients with any one of 86 metabolic disorders. Funded originally by the National Institute of Child Health and Human Development, MIN currently receives most of its support from pharmaceutical companies. Through MIN, an investigator doing research on a particular disease can locate other investigators doing related research. Names of patients are not included in the registry and requests for investigator-to-investigator contact are reviewed by a scientific advisory board.

A major concern of the Task Force is that as tests to diagnose and, in many cases, to predict, rare diseases are developed, data will not be systematically compiled on their clinical, as well as analytical validity. **A comprehensive system to collect data on rare diseases must be established.** As discussed in chapter 2, the Centers for Disease Control and Prevention (CDC) can and should play

---

[a]No numerical definition was given because of the uncertainty regarding the profitability of medical devices; some may be extremely expensive, yielding substantial returns on a small number of sales, while others may be in much greater demand but unable to earn enough revenue to justify their commercial development. (Personal communication, Emery J. Sturniolo, Office of Product Development, FDA, February 26, 1996.)

a role in coordinating data collection from multiple sources to facilitate the review of new genetic tests, particularly for rare diseases. Multiple sources will almost always be needed to validate tests for rare diseases. CDC and ORD should work closely to develop the appropriate data-gathering and monitoring systems to assess the validity of genetic tests for rare diseases.

Finding Information on the Interpretation of Clinical Findings

Some rare genetic diseases present with unusual symptoms or signs, making diagnosis relatively easy for knowledgeable physicians. Many rare inherited metabolic disorders present with commonly encountered problems for which the usual explanation is *not* a rare disease.[5] When the clinical problem persists or recurs despite treatment, health care providers must be aware that a rare disease could be the explanation. Prompt recognition can often save the patient's life by leading to initiation of effective therapy before irreversible damage occurs. Many of these metabolic disorders appear in infants and children; early diagnosis can alert the parents to their risk of having another affected child. Several tests can be used predictively for prenatal diagnosis. Carrier testing in collateral relatives is often possible.

Unfortunately, the diagnosis of rare diseases is often delayed. One reason for the delay is inaccessibility of information. **Physicians who encounter patients with symptoms and signs of rare genetic diseases should have access to accurate information that will enable them to include such diseases in their differential diagnosis, to know where to turn for assistance in clinical and laboratory diagnosis, and to locate laboratories that test for rare diseases.** The commonly encountered symptoms and signs with which rare diseases present and the process of evaluating them should be taught to medical students and residents. It would be too much to expect health care providers to retain

Delays in diagnosis of rare diseases. "Physicians are often unfamiliar with the vague and confusing symptoms of rare diseases. Almost one-third of the [801] patients surveyed indicated it took from 1 to 5 years to obtain a diagnosis, and one in seven went undiagnosed for 6 years or more. Only half of the respondents report receiving a diagnosis less than 1 year after first visiting a doctor."--Report of the National Commission on Orphan Diseases, U.S. Department of Health and Human Services, Public Health Service, Office of the Assistant Secretary of Health, February 1989, p. xiv.

information on all the unusual presentations, but they should be taught where to seek information. Although textbooks and medical journals are the classical starting points, and referrals to specialists may help, computerized databases in which a user could search by the patient's presenting finding would be more expeditious and effective. Most available information is organized by disease, not by presenting findings. The National Organization of Rare Diseases, Inc. (NORD) publishes The Physician's Guide to Rare Diseases, which includes an atlas of visual diagnostic signs. NORD also maintains the rare disease database containing entries on over 1,100 rare diseases. The database is logically organized by a description of the disorder, symptoms, causes, affected population, related disorders, diagnostic procedures, status of treatment (investigational or standard of care), resource referral for further information and support, and references from peer-reviewed medical literature. The database is available on the World Wide Web at http://www.nord-rdb.com/~orphan.

Although primarily providing information to researchers, the Metabolic Information Network can provide information to physicians on over 200 metabolic disorders.

Once diagnoses are made, patients and/or their families often want written information about the diseases. In a survey of 270 physicians conducted about 10 years ago, 42% were unable to find printed information to distribute to their patients with rare diseases.[1] NORD's database on rare diseases has since been made available to consumers. NORD also maintains a Patient Services Department, one of whose functions is to help affected individuals and families in need of accessing services. The Department also maintains a confidential patient registry.

Information about individual disorders, particularly for consumers, is also available through individual genetic support organizations, which can be located through NORD (Washington, DC) or the Alliance of Genetic Support Groups (Chevy Chase, Maryland).

Finding Clinical Diagnostic Laboratories

Because of the rarity of many diseases, only one or a few laboratories in the United States, or the world, accurately perform tests for them. This raises the problem of how physicians caring for patients will be able to identify these laboratories in time to benefit patients who present with acute illness.

The Helix Directory of Medical Genetics Laboratories, supported by the National Library of Medicine, lists approximately 300 laboratories that perform tests on over 480 genetic diseases. Helix began by listing laboratories performing DNA-based tests including fluorescent in situ hybridization (FISH), but will extend to biochemical tests in the future. As of July 1997, Helix has 4,500 registered users and receives 150 requests per day. (Personal communication, Maxine L. Covington, Helix Directory Manager, July 23, 1997) Helix provides information by phone and fax, but it is encouraging inquiries via the World Wide Web at http://www.hslib.washington.edu/helix. As many of the laboratories entered in the database do not want to be contacted directly by patients, passwords for entry to the database are available only to health care providers. Consequently, Helix is not listed in NORD's databases.

Through ORD's database on clinical research studies, physicians can get help in the diagnosis of patients in whom they suspect particular rare diseases. **To maintain and expand its database, ORD should identify laboratories worldwide that perform tests for rare genetic diseases, the methodology employed, and whether the tests they provide are in the investigational stage, or are being used for clinical diagnosis and decision making.**

Need for Coordination

The Task Force is concerned that there might be some unnecessary duplication of effort in compiling databases while, at the same time, some diseases or laboratories offering tests will not be included. In addition to the databases mentioned so far, several other organizations, including the Alliance of Genetic Support Groups, some of its member organizations, and other independent genetic disease interest groups maintain databases and, in some cases, patient registries. The American Academy of Pediatrics provides information periodically on newborn screening and other disorders. The Society for Inherited Metabolic Disorders is compiling information for providers about diagnostic evaluations of rare disorders, and ACMG is developing databases on tests that should be used to diagnose specific disorders. **In order to avoid redundancy and to use the**

expertise of these organizations more efficiently, NIH should assign its Office of Rare Diseases (ORD) the task of coordinating these efforts and provide ORD with sufficient funds to fulfill the Task Force's recommendations on rare diseases. ORD should periodically report to the proposed Secretary's Advisory Committee on the status of these activities. With CDC playing a greater role in genetics, it should be closely involved in activities in this area.

ENSURING CONTINUED AVAILABILITY OF TESTS FOR RARE DISEASES

The clinical diagnostic tests for some rare diseases are available only from laboratories that are primarily engaged in research. Some of these laboratories perform clinical tests at no cost to the patient and with the primary purpose of furthering their own research. This raises two questions: First, what happens to the availability of the test for clinical diagnostic purposes when the laboratory (or laboratories) performing the assay ceases to do so because it switches to other research projects or for other reasons? Second, as discussed in the concluding section, how can the quality of clinical test performance be assured in laboratories engaged primarily in research?

Research laboratories that were offering genetic tests for rare diseases will cease performing them as they complete their investigations and move on to other areas of interest. This is particularly a problem for the continued availability of clinical tests when only one research laboratory performed the test. It is not unlikely, however, that as progress on a given rare disease is made, all of the research laboratories offering tests will move on to solve other problems.

The Task Force considered the transitioning problem at great length. It rejected the possibility of creating central or regional laboratories that could perform a wide range of tests for rare diseases because assembling the necessary expertise for performing and interpreting all of the tests under one roof would be difficult or impossible. For the same reason, it rejected transfer of these tests to large mega-test commercial laboratories that might be willing to add on tests for rare diseases if they could cover costs. The Task Force also considered whether agencies funding research that included the development and offering of tests for rare diseases should be asked to allocate a small part of the grant or contract they awarded to enable the investigator to transfer the test to a service laboratory just before funding for the research terminated. This might discourage investigators from applying for grants if they were reluctant to take on this responsibility. Agencies funding research might also be reluctant to use funds to establish service activities. They might also have concerns about the quality of the tests being offered as a service.

The Task Force is not convinced that the transitioning problem is insurmountable. One possibility is that a laboratory that was offering genetic tests as part of its research, but on which clinical decisions were being made, procure CLIA certification (see below) and serve as a service laboratory, recovering its costs for the test by instituting charges for it. Another possibility is for the research laboratory to transfer the testing capabilities to the clinical diagnostic laboratory in its institution. The proximity of the expert investigator could facilitate a smooth transition and ensure the test would be performed and interpreted properly. A third possibility is that the test be transferred to a research laboratory elsewhere that is willing to perform the test as a service. In this case, mechanisms are needed to ensure that providers know where to obtain the test. Whichever

81

alternative is adopted, the test should undergo some form of external review before transition to a service.

The NIH Office of Rare Diseases should have the lead responsibility in ensuring the continued availability of safe and effective tests for rare diseases when it learns that a test will cease being offered. Funds to enable it to accomplish this task should be available. Laboratories should notify ORD about impending cessation of their testing so that provisions for a transition to other laboratories can be made. ORD should, in turn, notify other laboratories when a demonstrably safe and effective genetic test ceases to be available and make every effort to get another laboratory to perform it. If this fails, ORD should notify the other organizations with whom it coordinates, as well as the proposed Secretary's Advisory Committee.

ENSURING THE QUALITY OF GENETIC TESTS FOR RARE DISEASES

Neither the clinical nor the laboratory diagnosis of rare inherited diseases is easy. If clinicians do not mention the possibility of a rare disorder when they order clinical laboratory tests, the laboratory might not test for them. Clinical laboratories, too, might misinterpret abnormal findings, often neglecting rare disorders in favor of more common situations, such as poisoning. Some clinical laboratories do not have the equipment or expertise to diagnose a rare disorder, but clinicians might not realize it. (That is one reason why directories of qualified laboratories, as will be discussed further, are so important.) Many rare disorders will be diagnosed only by special laboratories accustomed to looking for rare diseases and having the equipment and expertise to do so.

Some genetic tests for rare diseases have been developed in research laboratories under grants. **In accordance with current law, the Task Force recommends that any laboratory performing any genetic test on which clinical diagnostic and/or management decisions are made should be certified under CLIA. Research laboratories that are not currently providing genetic test results to providers or patients but that plan to do so in the future must register under CLIA.** Once a laboratory registers, it does not have to wait for a survey (see chapter 3) before performing clinical tests.

Some research laboratories have complained of the difficulty and expense of obtaining CLIA approval for tests that constitute a small part of their activity and will only be performed occasionally. A laboratory performing 2,000 or fewer tests a year can register for $100 and obtain certification for $300 (including onsite inspection for its first 2 years.)[b]

---

[b]Charges can be higher if an exempt State or a deemed private organization conducts the survey (see chapter 3).

Errors in clinical laboratory diagnosis of rare diseases. A 3-month-old child was brought by his parents to an emergency department because he had become progressively unresponsive and was breathing rapidly. An independent clinical laboratory reported that the infant had a large amount of ethylene glycol (antifreeze) in his blood. Because the parents could not account for the infant's exposure to this toxic substance, he was placed in protective custody with foster parents, but the mother had visiting privileges. About 8 weeks later, the foster parents brought the infant to the emergency department when his problem recurred. This time, two laboratories independently claimed that ethylene glycol was elevated in the infant's blood. The infant's condition deteriorated and he died 3 days after admission to the hospital. The biologic mother was arrested and charged with first-degree murder. While in prison awaiting trial, the mother delivered a second child who was placed in foster care. Two weeks later, this infant became unresponsive with rapid breathing. The baby was admitted to a different hospital than its older sibling. A diagnosis of a rare inherited metabolic disease--methylmalonic acidemia--was promptly made and the infant started on appropriate therapy. Analysis of the younger sibling's blood for ethylene glycol showed that the abnormal metabolite could be distinguished from it. The mother was exonerated. A sample of blood to which the abnormal metabolite had been added was sent to a third independent laboratory. It, too, reported, erroneously, that the blood contained a large amount of ethylene glycol.[6]

In an accompanying report, an unrelated infant had recurrent symptoms similar to those described above. It was not until the third episode that blood and urine were obtained when the infant was acutely ill. They revealed ethylene glycol (but no methylmalonic acid or related metabolites). Ethylene glycol was also detected in two bottles of formula intended for consumption by the infant. A babysitter might have been responsible for the poisoning but the evidence was insufficient to indict.[7]

The Task Force recognizes the important contribution that research laboratories make to clinical testing, particularly for rare diseases. The type of skills that are needed for research, including a willingness to modify experimental conditions, are not necessarily the skills for maintaining the quality of a service laboratory, in which consistency of performance ensures reliability. **Research laboratories that provide physicians with results of genetic tests, which may be used for clinical decision making, must validate their tests and be subject to the same internal and external review as other clinical laboratories. Nevertheless, the proposed genetics subcommittee of CLIAC should consider developing regulatory language under the proposed genetics specialty that is less stringent, but does not sacrifice quality for laboratories that only occasionally and in small volume perform tests whose results are made available to health care providers or patients.[c]**

---

[c]Accommodations have been made for rare, genetic disease testing within the New York State Department of Health laboratory permit process. Physicians must obtain approval for tests performed on New York State residents in laboratories not approved by the State. One situation in which the State grants such approval is if the noncertified laboratory is the only one available to provide a needed test. In granting

Of great concern to the Task Force, discussed at length in chapter 3, is whether certification under CLIA will ensure the quality of genetic tests, particularly those for rare genetic diseases. The creation of a subspecialty of genetics under CLIA will greatly improve the situation. Many tests for rare disorders are biochemical. The quality of performance of these tests would be ensured if they were included under a genetics specialty.

Directories of laboratories that perform tests for rare genetic diseases should indicate whether or not the laboratory is CLIA-certified and whether it has satisfied other quality assessment and proficiency assessments, such as those provided by CAP and ACMG. Directors of these laboratories are encouraged to participate in these programs or other programs of at least comparable quality that may be established.

The Task Force is concerned that third-party payers, including managed care organizations will not recognize that tests for rare diseases can only be performed in certain highly-specialized laboratories. Patients will be misdiagnosed and harmed unless these laboratories are used. The Society for Inherited Metabolic Diseases is preparing a list of laboratories qualified to perform tests for several rare diseases. The Helix database should also indicate whether the laboratories listed in it are CLIA-registered and/or certified. When the proposed genetics specialty is established, the directories should indicate whether the laboratory performing genetic tests is certified in that specialty or the appropriate subspecialty.

---

permission, the State makes it clear that it cannot attest to the quality of the laboratory performing the test and requests that the physician indicate that to the patient. (State of New York, Department of Health. Genetic Testing Quality Assurance Program: Testing in Laboratories That Do Not Hold Permit. March 1996)

REFERENCES

1. National Commission on Orphan Diseases: Report of the National Commission on Orphan Diseases. 1989;(Abstract)

2. Public Law 97-414: 1995;U.S.C. Sec 360aa et:(Abstract)

3. Public Law 100-290: Orphan Drug Amendments of 1988. 1995;U.S.C. Sec 360cc(a):(Abstract)

4. Public Law: Safe Medical Devices Act of 1990. 1995;U.S.C. Sec 360j(m):(Abstract)

5. Holtzman NA: Rare diseases, common problems: Recognition and management. *Pediatrics* 1978;62:1056-1060.

6. Shoemaker JD, Lynch RE, Hoffmann JW, Sly WS: Misidentification of propionic acid as ethylene glycol in a patient with methylmalonic acidemia. *Journal of Pediatrics* 1992;120:417-421.

7. Woolf AD, Wynshaw-Boris A, Rinaldo P, Levy HL: Intentional infantile ethylene glycol poisoning presenting as an inherited metabolic disorder. *Journal of Pediatrics* 1992;120:421-424.

CHAPTER 6. SUMMARY AND CONCLUSIONS

The Task Force recommends that the Secretary of Health and Human Services appoint an advisory committee on genetic testing to be instrumental in implementing the recommendations of this Task Force. The advisory committee or its designate should establish a system for determining which genetic tests require stringent scrutiny. If a test is likely to be used to predict future disease in healthy people, it is a candidate for stringent scrutiny, but not all predictive tests will necessarily require such scrutiny and other criteria are needed as well.

The Task Force wishes to highlight the following recommendations and to indicate the organizations primarily responsible for facilitating them:

(1) **Protocols for the development of genetic tests that can be used predictively must receive the approval of an institutional review board (IRB) when subject identifiers are retained and when the intention is to make the test readily available for clinical use.** OPRR in cooperation with the proposed Secretary's Advisory Committee is primarily responsible.

(2) **Test developers must submit their validation and clinical utility data to external review as well as to interested professional organizations in order to permit informed decisions about routine use.** Independent review should take place at both the local level (e.g., academic center or company), and at the national level by professional societies, consensus panels, Federal agencies and other organizations, before new tests become available for noninvestigational clinical use. The proposed Secretary's Advisory Committee should coordinate national efforts.

(3) **The Task Force urges the newly created genetics subcommittee of the Clinical Laboratory Improvement Advisory Committee to consider the creation of a specialty of genetics that would encompass all predictive tests that satisfy criteria for stringent scrutiny. If only a subspecialty for DNA/RNA-based tests is feasible, the subcommittee must then address how to ensure the quality of laboratories performing nonDNA/RNA predictive genetic tests.** The agencies primarily responsible for administering CLIA, HCFA and CDC, should take the lead in implementing this recommendation.

(4) **The Task Force encourages the development of genetics curricula in medical school and residency training. In addition to these basic curricula, each specialty involved with the care of patients with disorders with significant genetic components should design relevant curricula for continuing education in genetics. Schools of nursing, public health, and social work need to strengthen and expand their training programs in genetics.** The newly created National Coalition for Health Professional Education in Genetics should greatly facilitate improving professional education in genetics.

(5) **Hospitals and managed care organizations should request evidence of competence before permitting providers to order predictive stringent scrutiny genetic tests or to counsel about them.** Implementation is at the local level. If accrediting organizations include a review of the management of selected genetic tests as part of their accreditation, there will be greater stimulus for local organizations to ensure quality.

(6) **Physicians who encounter patients with symptoms and signs of rare genetic diseases should have access to accurate information that will enable them to include such diseases in their differential diagnosis, to know where to turn for assistance in clinical and laboratory diagnosis, and to locate laboratories that test for rare diseases. The quality of laboratories**

providing tests for rare diseases must be assured, and a comprehensive system to collect data on rare diseases must be established. The NIH Office of Rare Diseases should play a coordinating role. The genetics subcommittee of CLIAC should examine means of assuring the quality of laboratories performing tests for rare diseases.

These and the many other principles and recommendations of the Task Force presented herein will help ensure that genetic testing will be provided safely and effectively and that tests for rare diseases will be more widely available but used appropriately. The Task Force concludes that with implementation of these recommendations, genetic testing will continue to flourish.

APPENDIX 1. INDIVIDUALS AND ORGANIZATIONS WHO PROVIDED COMMENTS TO THE TASK FORCE

The following individuals and the organizations they either represent or which they listed for identification purposes responded to the Task Force's request for comments on its Interim Principles (distributed on request; Task Force's website at http://www.med.jhu.edu/tfgtelsi) and/or on its Proposed Recommendations (Fed. Reg. 1997; 62:4539-4547; Task Force's website). The list includes people who testified at the Task Force's public hearing on its Interim Principles on April 30, 1996, and who submitted written comments on the Interim Principles, the Proposed Recommendations, or both.

Joann Adair, R.N.
Commonwealth of Pennsylvania
  Department of Health

Nilofer Nina Ahmad, Ph.D.
Wills Eye Hospital

Leslie Alexandre, Dr. P.H.
OncorMed

William Audeh, M.D.
Cedars-Sinai Medical Center

Robert C. Baumiller
Xavier University

Deborah Blacker, M.D., Sc.D.
American Psychiatric Association

Ann Boldt, M.S., C.G.C.
National Society of Genetic Counselors

David T. Bonk
Bristol-Myers Squibb Company

Barbara A. Brenner
Breast Cancer Action

M. Desmond Burke
American Society of Clinical Pathologists

Peter H. Byers, M.D.
American Board of Medical Genetics

Michael Camilleri, M.D.
C. Christopher Hook, M.D.
Mayo Foundation

Robert C. Cefalo, M.D., Ph.D.
American Board of Obstetrics and
  Gynecology

Ellen Wright Clayton
Vanderbilt University

Jordan J. Cohen, M.D.
Association of American Medical Colleges

Anne Marie Comeau, Ph.D.
New England Regional Newborn
  Screening Program

Celeste M. Condit
The University of Georgia

Donald R. Coustan, M.D.
J.E. Ferguson
Society of Perinatal Obstetricians

Jo Linder-Crow, Ph.D.
American Psychological Association

Shelly Cummings
University of Chicago Medical Center

George C. Cunningham, M.D., M.P.H.
State of California - Health and Welfare
  Agency

Mary E. Davidson
Joan Burns
Alliance of Genetic Support Groups

Barbara A. DeBuono, M.D., M.P.H.
State of New York, Dept. of Health

Laurence M. Demers, Ph.D.
American Association for Clinical
  Chemistry, Inc.

Rochelle Diamond
National Organization of Gay & Lesbian
  Scientists and Technical Professionals,
  Incorporated

Joyce Dolcourt
Mountain States Regional Genetic Services
  Network

Louis J. Elsas, II, M.D.
Council of Regional Network for Genetic
  Services

Ray Erickson
Consumer

Carolyn D. Farrell, M.S., C.N.P., C.G.C.
Roswell Park Cancer Institute

James E. Ferguson, II, M.D.
Member of the Board, Society of Perinatal
  Obstetricians

Donna G. B. Getz
Consumer

Lynn Godmilow
University of Pennsylvania School of
  Medicine

Alan Goldhammer, Ph.D.
Biotechnology Industry Organization

Julian Gordon
Abbott Labs

Margaret L. Gulley, M.D.
Association for Molecular Pathology

Barbara Handelin, Ph.D.
Handelin Associates

Janet E. Haskell
Myriad Genetic Laboratories, Inc.

P. Hathaway, M.D.
M. C. Sullivan, R.N., J. D.
R. Flanigan, Ph.D.
The Midwest Bioethics Center

Elliott D. Hillback
Genzyme

Joseph Q. Jarvis, M.D.
Mountain State Regional Genetics Services
  Network

John P. Johnson, M.D.
Mountain State Regional Genetics Services
  Network

Haig H. Kazazian, M.D.
University of Pennsylvania

Charles Kull
Consumer

Lisa S. Lehmann, M.D.
Dana-Farber Cancer Institute

Bill Letson
State of Wyoming Department of Health

Sue Levi-Pearl
National Tourette Association

Allen Lichter, M.D.
American Society of Clinical Oncology

Casey Maddren
Consumer

Mary Mahowald
University of Chicago

Mamie Malo
Consumer

Susan Panny, M.D.
Maryland Department of Health and Mental
  Hygiene

Kenneth A. Pass, Ph.D.
State of New York Department of Health

Frances A. Pitlick, Ph.D.
Biochemist

Beth A. Pletcher, M.D.
Franklin Desposito, M.D.
American Academy of Pediatrics

George Poste
Tadataka Yamada, M.D.
SmithKline Beecham Pharmaceuticals

Reed Edwin Pyeritz, M.D., Ph.D.
American College of Medical Genetics

Kenneth A. Pass, Ph.D.
State of New York Department of Health

Frances A. Pitlick, Ph.D.
Biochemist

Beth A. Pletcher, M.D.
Franklin Desposito, M.D.
American Academy of Pediatrics

George Poste
Tadataka Yamada, M.D.
SmithKline Beecham Pharmaceuticals

Reed Edwin Pyeritz, M.D., Ph.D.
American College of Medical Genetics

Cathie S. Ragovin, M.D.
Massachusetts Breast Cancer Coalition

Pamela J. Reidy
Association of Women's Health
  Obstetric and Neonatal Nurses

Margaret "Wendy" Ricker, Ed.D.
Consumer

David Rimoin, M.D., Ph.D.
American College of Medical Genetics

Allen Roses, M.D.
Duke University Medical Center

Mark A. Rothstein
University of Houston Law Center

Peter T. Rowley, M.D.
University of Rochester Medical Center

Lester B. Salans
Sandoz Pharmaceuticals Corporation

Jerry Schenken, M.D.
The Pathology Center

P. John Seward, M.D.
American Medical Association

Larry J. Shapiro, M.D.
The American Society of Human Genetics

Karen Snow, Ph.D.
Mayo Clinic

David A. Sobel, Ph.D.
Confidentiality Matters

Peter Somani, M.D., Ph.D.
Ohio Department of Health

Kathryn Sudduth, C.L.Sp.(C.G.)
Association of Cytogenetic Technologists

Herbert S. Waxman, M.D., F.A.C.P.
American College of Physicians

Joan O. Weiss, M.S.W.
Alliance of Genetic Support Groups

Benjamin S. Wilfond, M.D.
The University of Arizona Health Sciences
  Center

Philip R. Wyatt, M.D., Ph.D.
North York General Hospital - Genetics

Raymond C. Zastrow, M.D.
College of American Pathologists

Stanley Zinberg, M.D., M.S., F.A.C.O.G.
The American College of Obstetricians &
  Gynecologists

APPENDIX 2. RESPONSE OF THE TASK FORCE TO THE FOOD AND DRUG ADMINISTRATION'S PROPOSED RULE ON ANALYTE SPECIFIC REAGENTS

Background

Analyte specific reagents (ASR's) are chemicals, including DNA probes, that are the active ingredients of tests for diagnosing, or predicting risks of, diseases in humans. These reagents can be purchased by manufacturers of tests that are approved by FDA and also by clinical laboratories for use in in-house ("home brew") tests, for which FDA does not require approval. By law, ASR's are medical devices, but FDA had done little to regulate them.

On January 22, 1996 FDA sought the approval of its Immunology Devices Panel for requiring manufacturers of ASR's to register with FDA and provide the agency with a list of the ASR's they are supplying to laboratories for use in developing tests. FDA also asked the panel to approve requiring the manufacturers of ASR's to follow good manufacturing practices (GMP), as defined by FDA, as well as other general controls, including restrictions on the distribution and labeling of ASR's, and to report adverse events that may have been due to ASR's. The panel approved these proposals, including limiting the distribution of ASR's to laboratories certified as high complexity under CLIA (see Chapter 3). The panel recommended that when reporting results from in-house tests using ASR's, laboratories had to include a disclaimer that the test had not been reviewed by FDA. The panel also recommended that manufacturers could not make analytical or clinical performance claims for their ASR. FDA also sought the panel's approval on classifying most ASR's as class I devices, but exempting them from the premarket notification requirements of section 510(k) of the Food, Drug, and Cosmetic Act. (Class I devices are those for which general controls, including registration and GMP, are sufficient to assure safety and effectiveness of their intended use.) The panel approved, but recommended that tests to predict genetic disease in healthy or apparently healthy individuals be added to those ASR's that should be placed into class II or class III. (Class II devices require special controls and class III devices are those in which neither general nor special controls provide reasonable assurance of safety and effectiveness and require premarket approval from FDA.)

On March 14, 1996, FDA published its proposed recommendations for ASR's, responding to the Immunology Devices Panel comments.[a] In its proposed recommendations, FDA did not place predictive genetic tests in class II or class III. However, it invited "comments on the full range of options available to regulate ASR's intended for use in human genetic testing: From regulating these ASR's as class I exempt products to regulating them as class III devices subject to premarket approval." In accord with the panel's recommendation FDA required manufacturers of ASR's to include on the label, "Analytical and performance characteristics are not established." It invited comments on whether in-house tests using ASR's should carry warnings to those who ordered them, but it did not include such a warning in its proposed recommendations.

The following letter was in response to FDA's proposed recommendations.

---

[a]Medical devices; classification/reclassification; restricted devices; analyte specific reagents. Federal Register 61(51):10484–10489. March 14, 1996.

550 N. Broadway, Suite 511
Baltimore, Maryland 21205
(410) 955-7894
Fax (410) 955-0241

June 11, 1996

Dockets Management Branch (HFA-305)
Food and Drug Administration
12420 Parklawn Dr.
Rm. 1-23
Rockville, MD 20857

RE: Docket #96N-0082-Medical Devices; Classification/Reclassification; Restricted Devices; Analyte Specific Reagents

The attached document was drafted by a subcommittee of the Task Force on Genetic Testing including Neil Holtzman, Michael Watson, Patricia Murphy, Stephen Goodman and Victoria Odesina and represents a majority consensus opinion. The draft prepared by the subcommittee was circulated to the entire Task Force. A majority of voting members supported the document, but approval was not unanimous. Additionally, the document does not necessarily represent the points of view of the organizations represented by those drafting the document nor of the organizations represented by others on the Task Force.

As to substance, a minority opinion was held that the onus should not be on the manufacturer of the product used in "home brew" assays, but rather that alternative or new approaches to assuring that ASR's are used appropriately by the laboratories building those tests were required.

The Task Force on Genetic Testing was convened to review genetic testing in the United States and make recommendations to ensure the development of safe and effective genetic tests, their delivery in laboratories of assured quality, and their appropriate use by health care providers and consumers. The Task Force is responding to FDA's solicitation of comments on the regulation of analyte specific reagents (ASR's) intended for use in human genetic testing. We applaud FDA for establishing labeling requirements for ASR's. Despite the greater assurance of product integrity that good manufacturing practice (GMP) oversight and the proposed labeling provides, the Task Force finds it inadequate for genetic tests for three reasons. First, certain intended uses of genetic tests engender

94

questions of safety and effectiveness that require a greater level of control. Second, the proposal omits from regulation clinical testing laboratories that make their ASR's "in-house" for "home brew" tests (to use FDA's terminology). Third, restricting the sale of ASR's to high complexity laboratories as defined under the Clinical Laboratory Improvement Amendments of 1988 (CLIA-'88), as FDA proposes, does not afford adequate assurance of safety and effectiveness. We will discuss each of these in turn.

Intended uses of genetic tests

Genetic tests can be used clinically to predict disease risks, identify carriers, diagnose disease, monitor progression of disease and response to therapy, and suggest the prognosis. The same genetic test can be used for more than one of these purposes. Some tests provide information about acquired as well as inherited disease. For instance, tests for mutations in the p53 gene can be used to predict and diagnose inherited cancer (Li-Fraumeni syndrome) with high predictability, as well as to assist in staging particular types of acquired tumors, and to identify the category of environmental mutagens responsible for the tumor.

It is predictive uses of tests for inherited disorders that are of great concern to the Task Force. These tests raise complex psychosocial issues. Moreover, their clinical validity may be difficult to establish and their sensitivity and predictive value may not be high. Nor, in some instances, have the benefits they confer been proven. Consequently, test interpretation requires training and experience in human genetics and genetic counseling.

Positive test results for germline mutations in common complex disorders do not often carry as high predictive values as observed in single-gene (Mendelian) disorders like the Li-Fraumeni syndrome. In some instances, frequently occurring "normal" alleles (polymorphisms) have been associated with common diseases, such as insulin-dependent diabetes mellitus (non-asp57 HLA DQ beta alleles) and Alzheimer disease (Apolipoprotein e4 allele), but many, if not most, people with these alleles will not develop the specific diseases.

Predictive testing in the general population (screening) has a greater chance of clinical false positive test results than testing in high risk families. The predictive value of a positive (PVP) test for an inherited susceptibility mutation in the BRCA1 gene in healthy individuals who do not have a family history of breast cancer (*i.e.*, screening) may be considerably lower than the PVP of approximately 85 percent observed in women from high risk families.

Because of allelic diversity, and new mutations in X-linked and dominant disorders, negative test results for single-gene disorders do not always exclude the presence of a disease-related allele. Even when the predictive value of positive and negative test results is high, as in families with the Li-Fraumeni syndrome, psychosocial concerns of those tested can be great.

For many genetic disorders, safe and effective interventions have not been established, so healthy individuals with positive test results face considerable uncertainty about what course of action is

95

best. For instance, the benefits and risks of mammography in asymptomatic young women found to have an inherited BRCA1 susceptibility mutation, or of prophylactic mastectomy, oophorectomy, or chemoprophylaxis are not currently known.

The Task Force is of the opinion that a predictive genetic test should not be available on any but an investigative basis until information on its clinical validity and clinical utility is available or until detailed protocols for gathering this information are in place. This has been accomplished, for instance, in tests for mutations in the RET oncogene that are highly predictive of multiple endocrine neoplasia type 2. Preliminary data in predictive tests for other disorders, such as the Apolipoprotein e4 test for Alzheimer disease, have not been convincing. By limiting regulation of ASR's used for predictive genetic tests to the labeling requirements in proposed paragraph (e) of 21 CFR part 809.10, FDA will encourage the use of such tests without collection of the requisite data to ensure their safety and effectiveness.

In regulating *in vitro* diagnostics, FDA relies heavily on the intended use of the device as stated on the manufacturer's proposed label. This should hold true for predictive genetic tests as well. The Task Force is of the opinion that ASR's capable of being used for predictive genetic tests, such as human DNA probes or primers, should be excepted from Sec. 864.4020 (b)(1) of the proposed rule and added to the categories listed in Sec. 864.4020 (b)(2). Human DNA is not the only category of ASR's capable of being used in genetic tests. Assays for enzymes and other proteins, which may employ ASR's, can yield predictive information for both carriers and apparently healthy affected individuals. It is also likely that monoclonal antibodies raised against specific proteins will be used to test for genetic diseases. Consequently, it accomplishes little to exclude human nucleic acids from the definition of ASR's, as proposed by the Immunology Devices Panel.

Because of the wide range of ASR's that could be used for predictive genetic testing, FDA must, in the opinion of the Task Force, develop policies to determine which categories of ASR's could be used for predictive genetic testing. To assist it in this task, FDA should convene a Genetic Test Devices Panel under its Medical Devices Advisory Committee. This panel could establish criteria for determining whether an ASR could be used for predictive genetic testing. When such a determination is made, this panel could advise FDA on the classification of the ASR.

An alternative approach, which is less enforceable and, consequently, less desirable in the opinion of the Task Force, is to require manufacturers to label every ASR as "not for use in predictive genetic tests without the approval of FDA." As FDA knows, the labeling of reagents "for research use only" or "for investigative use only" has not precluded their use in routine clinical tests in humans. Similarly, there has been little control over off-label uses of many approved drugs and devices.

In-house testing

In the background to its proposal, FDA states that "at a future date" it may "reevaluate whether additional controls over the in-house tests" are needed. It further acknowledges such controls as "especially relevant. . . as testing for the presence of genes associated with cancer or dementing diseases becomes more widely available." Predictive genetic tests for breast and colon cancer and for Alzheimer disease are already available.

The Task Force is of the opinion that laboratories that use ASR's for in-house predictive genetic tests should establish safety and effectiveness of their tests before making them available on any but an investigative basis. The Task Force recognizes that the considerable time and expense that may be needed to determine safety and effectiveness could deter clinical laboratories from developing and providing genetic tests. FDA should consider how it can expedite assessments of safety and effectiveness of predictive genetic tests that are provided in-house. Until additional policies are established, the Task Force agrees with the Immunology Devices Panel's recommendation that "laboratories, when reporting results from in-house developed tests using ASR's, include a disclaimer ...." However, we would suggest that the disclaimer indicate that "This test has been developed in-house and analytically validated under the requirements of CLIA '88." Unless otherwise noted, the disclaimer should indicate that "the safety and effectiveness of the test have not been established."

Protection afforded under CLIA-'88

CLIA-'88 provides no authority for assessing either the clinical validity or utility of a test, although laboratories are required to demonstrate the analytical validity of tests they develop. Consequently, restricting the sale of ASR's to laboratories qualified for high complexity testing under CLIA-'88 will not ensure the safety and effectiveness of predictive genetic tests. Moreover, laboratories qualified for high complexity testing do not necessarily employ personnel with special training and/or experience in genetics, which is crucial if the laboratory is to provide an adequate and appropriate interpretation of the results of predictive tests.

The performance of predictive genetic tests should be restricted to laboratories with expertise in genetics and demonstrated proficiency in genetic testing. Unfortunately, there is no genetics specialty under CLIA. Although one is in place for cytogenetics, none exists for molecular genetics or biochemical genetics. Nor does the Department of Health and Human Services (HHS) through the Health Care Financing Administration, which administers CLIA-'88, require that laboratories performing genetic tests participate in proficiency testing programs, which already exist, for several categories of genetic tests. With a genetics specialty under CLIA, personnel requirements for laboratories performing genetic tests could be established, as could requirements for proficiency testing. Having a specialty would not, however, address the Task Force's concerns about the clinical validity of genetic tests.

Summary

The following reflect our primary concerns and recommendations about the ASR proposal.

> * Genetic tests have many intended uses. When an ASR has the capability of predicting inherited disease in healthy or apparently healthy individuals it must not receive a Class I

97

classification, exempt from premarket notification. If, however, FDA rejects this recommendation it should require manufacturers to include on the label the statement: "Not for use in predictive genetic tests without the approval of FDA."

* FDA should establish a Genetic Test Devices Panel under its Medical Devices Advisory Committee. Such a panel could assist FDA in determining whether an ASR could be used for predictive genetic testing. When such a determination is made, this panel could advise FDA on the classification of the ASR.

* FDA should consider how it can expedite assessments of safety and effectiveness of predictive genetic tests that are provided in-house. Until additional policies are established, the reporting of results of tests developed in-house should include the disclaimer that the test has been analytically validated under the requirements of CLIA-'88. Unless otherwise noted, it should be indicated that the safety and effectiveness of the test have not been established.

* Restricting the sale of ASR's to laboratories certified as high complexity laboratories under CLIA-'88 does not assure the safety and effectiveness of predictive genetic tests nor of most other tests for disorders with complex inheritance.

* A genetics specialty should be established under CLIA-'88. This would facilitate establishing personnel requirements for laboratories performing predictive genetic tests, as well as requirements for proficiency testing. Having a specialty would not, however, address the Task Force's concerns about the clinical validity of genetic tests.

With no provision for establishing the clinical validity of predictive genetic tests, and no assurance that laboratories performing predictive tests will do so, FDA's proposal on ASR's as it relates to predictive genetic tests, affords the public inadequate protection.

Task Force on Genetic Testing

APPENDIX 3. STATE OF THE ART OF GENETIC TESTING IN THE UNITED STATES: SURVEY OF BIOTECHNOLOGY COMPANIES AND NONPROFIT CLINICAL LABORATORIES AND INTERVIEWS OF SELECTED ORGANIZATIONS[a]

Neil A. Holtzman[b] and Stephen Hilgartner[c]

The survey and follow-up interviews described here were conducted to provide the Task Force on Genetic Testing with three types of information: the extent of genetic testing in the United States; the policies and practices of organizations engaged in such testing, and the opinions of officials of the organizations contacted concerning matters related to genetic testing.

For our survey, we defined genetic tests as "the analysis of human DNA, RNA, chromosomes, proteins, or other gene products to detect disease-related genotypes, mutations, or phenotypes, or karyotypes for clinical purposes. Such purposes include prediction of disease risks, identification of carriers, monitoring, diagnosis or prognosis, and establishing genetic identity, but do not include tests conducted purely for research."

METHODS

Survey Populations

A list of American biotechnology companies and molecular genetics and cytogenetics laboratories operated by nonprofit organizations was compiled from the Institute for Biotechnology Information (IBI) database, the Helix National Directory of DNA Diagnostic Laboratories, and the Association of Cytogenetic Technologists (ACT) International Cytogenetic Laboratory Directory. A few organizations not in these databases but known to us were added. Descriptors in the IBI and ACT databases enabled us to limit our mailing to organizations that were likely to be developing or providing new genetic test technologies.[d]

Survey Instrument

The questionnaire consisted of 26 questions, some with several parts, and most in multiple choice format. The major categories covered are shown in Table 1. Respondents' personal agreement or disagreement with six statements was sought, using a four point Likert scale.

---

[a]This paper was undertaken for the Task Force on Genetic Testing with support from the National Human Genome Research Institute (R01-HG00026). Preliminary survey results were presented to the Task Force on April 13, 1995. A summary of the interview findings was presented to the Task Force on March 17, 1997. The views expressed in this paper are those of the authors and do not necessarily reflect the views of the Task Force.

[b]The Johns Hopkins Medical Institutions, Baltimore, Maryland

[c]Cornell University, Ithaca, New York

[d]From the IBI database we selected U.S. companies listed under the following descriptors: biotech, diagnostics, chemical, new company, incomplete data, refused to respond to IBI's questionnaire. These companies also had to fit into one or more of the following biotechnology industry classifications: clinical human diagnostics, medical devices, testing/analytical services; biotechnology equipment, reagents or construction/engineering; bioseparations, research, therapeutics, vaccines, or consulting. From the ACT data base, we selected laboratories whose codes for work performed included: sister chromatid exchange, in situ hybridization (any type), molecular techniques, and mutagenicity testing. All of the laboratories in the Helix database were included.

The questionnaire was pilot tested with five officials from university-based clinical laboratories and biotechnology companies engaged in genetic testing activities and amended accordingly.

Survey

The questionnaire was initially mailed in December 1994 and January 1995. If we received no reply in a month despite reminders, we sent a short questionnaire, which consisted of four questions from the long questionnaire on genetic testing activities. If the organization did not return the short questionnaire, we telephoned the organization to collect the information. For cytogenetic laboratories we did not use a phone call followup.

Interview Sample

Organizations were selected for an in-depth interview from among those who completed the long version of the survey. We selected ten of them because we were aware of their activities and judged them to be significant players in genetic testing. Selection of the other companies was based on the following criteria: The company had to indicate on the survey that it:

(1) was either developing or providing tests for at least one of several complex disorders (Alzheimer's, breast cancer, colon cancer, diabetes, melanoma) or single-gene disorders (cystic fibrosis, fragile X, Huntington's disease, Marfan syndrome, muscular dystrophies, or neurofibromatosis I or II), and

(2) devoted more than 10 percent of its financial resources to either research and development (R& D) and/or marketing of genetic tests and expected more than 30 percent of its revenue over the next five years to be derived from genetic testing, or

(3) expected revenue of $1 million and a biotechnology R&D budget of more than $2 million (current fiscal year), or

(4) expected revenue of more than $2 million with more than 5 percent of that revenue deriving from biotechnology activities.

(Data for 3 and 4 were obtained from the IBI data base.)

Twelve companies met criteria 1 and 2 and an additional six met criteria 1 plus 3 and/or 4. Five of the ten firms that we selected on the basis of our personal knowledge of their activities met criterion 1, and of these, two met both 2 and 3 and/or 4, two met 2 only and one met 3 or 4 only.[e]

A letter requesting an interview was sent to the company official who completed the questionnaire.[f] We also conducted interviews at five laboratories engaged in genetic testing at not-for-profit academic centers or managed care organizations. These labs were selected if they were in a geographic area that we planned to visit to interview companies, and if the interview could be scheduled at the time of the visit.

Beyond the companies studied, we make no claims about the quantitative frequency of the activities documented below. Some of the results presented here are intended to provide a qualitative sense of current activities in genetic testing that we could not probe in the survey. Others corroborate and extend findings of the survey.

---

[e] On a sixth company we had insufficient data to determine whether it satisfied the criteria.

[f] The titles of the officials contacted varied. They were directors of research and development, medical directors, directors of genetics, or, at smaller companies, vice presidents or presidents.

The Interview

The interview covered four major topics: the history of the organization's efforts in genetic testing; its specific R&D programs and projects; its plans and policies regarding R&D, marketing, quality control, and regulatory issues; and the organization's policies and the respondent's views toward regulatory, policy, and ethical issues in genetic testing. All respondents were promised anonymity. Explicit refusals to answer particular questions occurred infrequently and were generally confined to certain lines of inquiry, such as queries about the volume of testing a company performs, which some respondents considered particularly sensitive.

RESPONSE RATES

Of the 594 biotechnology companies (BTCs) who were mailed questionnaires, 194 (32.7 percent) returned the long questionnaire and 267 (44.9 percent) returned the short questionnaire for a total response rate of 77.6 percent. Of 425 nonprofit organizations (NPOs) surveyed, 273 (64.2 percent) returned the long questionnaire and 80 (18.8 percent) returned the short questionnaire for a total response rate of 83 percent. Although the proportions of long and short questionnaires returned by molecular and cytogenetic NPOs did not differ, the response rate of molecular NPOs was higher than of cytogenetic NPOs (92 percent versus 75 percent). Except when these two classes of NPOs differ, the results are pooled.

Of the 28 companies selected, interviews were conducted at 25 between June 1995 and January 1997.[g] In 16 cases, one of us visited the company and conducted the interviews in person; in 8 cases, interviews were conducted by telephone. Most interviews lasted between 1 and 1.5 hours.[h] All five of the nonprofit organizations agreed to be interviewed. These interviews were all conducted in person.

RESULTS OF SURVEY

Companies Not Developing Tests

Twenty-nine BTCs who returned the long questionnaire said they had considered developing genetic test products or services, but decided not to. The following eight reasons were selected in descending order: not our area of expertise (9); regulatory hurdles (7); we lack a unique product angle (5); high costs (4); controversial area (4); patent issues (3); too competitive (2); and limited demand (2). Companies could list more than one reason. Four BTCs gave other reasons, three of which involved lack of complete technology.

---

[g]Three interviews were not conducted because: We were unable to schedule one; one company refused, and one was no longer operating. In one of the 25 companies interviewed, an audiotape recording failure prevented transcription of the interview. This company is not considered further in this report.

[h]The transcripts ranged from 5,100 to 18,000 words with an average length of 9,900 words.

Genetic Testing Activities

Almost nine-tenths of NPOs (316) and one-third of responding BTCs (147) were engaged in genetic testing activity. Table 2 provides a breakdown from the responses to both the long and short questionnaires. As virtually all of the NPOs are clinical laboratories, it is not surprising that they are predominantly engaged in service activities. Fifty-eight BTCs were developing or providing genetic tests (39.5 percent) and 89.5 (60.5 percent) were engaged in related activities.

The remaining analyses are limited to those organizations who completed the long questionnaire.

Among the 186 NPOs offering genetic testing services, 103 (55.3 percent) use tests developed in-house (home brews). Of the 23 BTCs providing such services, 11 (47.8 percent) use home brews.

Fifty-three BTCs and 212 NPOs reported developing or offering genetic tests for at least 1 of the 44 disorders listed in the questionnaire. These included three common complex disorders (Alzheimer's disease, breast cancer, hereditary nonpolyposis colon cancer (HNPCC)) and three of the most frequent single-gene disorders (cystic fibrosis, fragile X, muscular dystrophy). A significantly higher proportion of these 53 BTCs were developing or offering tests for the 3 complex disorders (64 percent) than for the 3 single gene disorders (47 percent). Only 22 percent of NPOs were developing or offering tests for the complex disorders (Table 3).

Among the 34 BTCs developing or offering tests for complex disorders, 13 (38 percent) were targeting particular populations, compared to only 3 of 47 NPOs (6 percent). Prenatal diagnosis was checked as an intended use for the three complex disorders by four BTCs (12 percent) and three NPOs (6 percent). Three companies said testing in children was an intended use for tests for breast cancer or HNPCC.

Patenting and Licensing

Not surprisingly, BTCs were almost four times more likely to hold patents, have patents pending, or say they would file patents than NPOs ((62 percent versus 16 percent); p < 0.0001). Among the 25 BTCs that were offering genetic test services, 14 (56 percent) had or expected to have licensing agreements with other organizations, as did 40 of 120 NPO (33 percent) molecular laboratories, and 13 of 111 cytogenetics laboratories (12 percent). The BTCs offering genetic test services were more likely to have licensing arrangements with academic institutions than with other companies (13 versus 9 BTCs), whereas the NPOs were more likely to have licensing arrangements with other companies (43 versus 12).

Assessment and External Review of New Tests

We were interested in how often organizations developing new tests assessed their reliability and/or validity prior to making them routinely available. Thirty-five of the 43 BTCs and 179 of the 223 NPOs who answered this question said they were involved in such assessments. Organizations conducting these assessments might have done so under an Institutional Review Board (IRB) protocol or under an investigational device exemption (IDE) from the Food and Drug Administration (FDA). However, of the 43 BTCs only 25 (58.1 percent) had ever submitted, or said they were likely to submit, protocols for any aspect of test development to an IRB and only 13 (30.2 percent) had ever contacted the FDA for reasons related to genetic test development. Among the 215 NPOs who answered this question. 132 (61.4 percent) had ever submitted or planned to submit to an IRB, but only 17 (17.9 percent) had ever contacted the FDA.

Table 4 displays the data on IRB submission and FDA contact by whether the organization was developing, currently offering, or both developing and offering tests. It was only among those BTCs and NPOs that were both developing and currently offering genetic tests that more than half submitted a protocol to an IRB. Organizations who were only developing genetic tests may have been at a very preliminary stage in their test development, one at which they would not be expected to go to either an IRB or the FDA. Organizations who were just offering but not developing may have acquired the tests from other organizations and not have needed to submit to an IRB or contact the FDA. In an effort to adjust for these possibilities, we examined IRB and FDA contact among the 14 BTCs and 95 NPOs who reported preparing their own probes, primers, enzymes or special chemicals for the genetic tests they currently offered. About three-fourths of both the BTCs and NPOs who had developed such "home brews" had either submitted to an IRB or contacted the FDA.

One reason that so few organizations had contacted the FDA may have been because most genetic tests being developed or marketed (by both BTCs and NPOs) are planned or offered as services rather than as tangible products, such as kits.[i] We, therefore, looked at FDA contact only for those organizations that reported developing or offering genetic test *kits*. Of the 23 BTCs developing genetic test kits and 1 marketing a kit, only 1 (4 percent) had obtained an investigational device exemption (IDE) from FDA and 6 (25 percent) had filed a premarket notification (510k). Only three NPOs were developing or marketing genetic test kits and only one had obtained an IDE. None of these BTCs or NPOs had filed a premarket approval application. Six BTCs and one NPO had other communication with FDA regarding genetic testing.

We also examined the reported external review of those organizations developing or offering tests for the three complex disorders. At the time of the survey all three were still regarded as investigational by several professional societies. Eighteen of the 81 organizations (22.2 percent) developing or already offering tests for these disorders had not filed nor do they plan to file with an IRB and 62 (76.5 percent) had not contacted the FDA. However, of the 11 organizations that are already providing tests, 10 had submitted to an IRB, and 2 had contact with FDA. We cannot say, however, whether the submissions or contacts were for testing for these three disorders.

Laboratory Quality

Table 5 describes some quality assurance activities of the respondent organizations that were offering genetic test services. Most were registered under the Clinical Laboratory Improvement Amendment 1988 (CLIA). At the time of the survey and to the present, no proficiency testing program is required of CLIA-certified laboratories. The College of American Pathologists and the American College of Medical Genetics jointly administer voluntary proficiency testing programs for several types of genetic tests.

As shown in Table 5, only 3 BTCs (11.1 percent) but 16 NPO molecular laboratories (16.5 percent) fail to participate in either a formal proficiency testing or an informal sharing of unknown samples.

---

[i]FDA has chosen not to regulate medical devices such as the chemicals and instruments that constitute diagnostic tests when the tests are marketed as services by clinical laboratories.

Targeting of Tests

Most organizations currently offering genetic tests aim their marketing at geneticists, genetic counselors and nongenetics medical specialists (Table 5). Significantly more BTCs than NPOs target managed care organizations. Many organizations also target primary care physicians but few market directly to patients or consumers.

Testing of Minors

Of laboratories offering genetic testing services who answered the question, 7 BTCs (28.0 percent) had restrictions on performing genetic tests for carrier status or adult-onset diseases in minors compared to 54 NPO molecular laboratories (57 percent) and 34 NPO cytogenetic laboratories (44 percent; $p < 02$).

Opinions of Individual Respondents

We asked respondents to indicate their personal agreement or disagreement with each of six statements on genetic testing (Table 6). On two statements, BTC and NPO personnel differed. A significantly higher percentage of BTC (20 percent) than NPO (6 percent) respondents personally agreed with the statement that "Most physicians can interpret genetic tests adequately...." A significantly higher percentage of BTC (53 percent) than NPO (39 percent) respondents thought that current CLIA policies "assure the quality of genetic test services." There was widespread agreement with the statement that "Some laboratories that offer genetic testing lack quality assurance programs" (84 percent). Seventy-three percent agreed with the statement that "FDA policies, or lack of policies, hinder the development of safe and effective genetic test kits or other products." There was considerable agreement that an industry-wide code would improve genetic services (85 percent of all respondents), and that additional laws or regulations are needed to ensure the privacy of genetic information (70 percent).

RESULTS OF INTERVIEWS

For analytic purposes, the organizations interviewed can be divided into three categories: providers of testing services, including five not-for-profit laboratories (n=15); developers of testing technology (n=9), who are creating or improving generic DNA technologies that are applicable to genetic testing services or kits; and gene discovery firms (n=2), who are working to identify new genes involved in human disease with the ultimate goal of using these genes as the basis of therapeutic and diagnostic products. The research and policies of these gene discovery companies, which emerged only in the 1990s, are beginning to play an important role in the arena of genetic testing. Three other companies proved, on interview, to be in adjacent markets and were not directly involved in genetic testing.

The Market for Genetic Tests

The companies engaged in testing activities operate in an extremely dynamic environment, frequently undergoing restructuring, forming new partnerships, embarking on new initiatives, or dropping projects. For example, one company, which had achieved some success in a generic DNA testing technology, partnered off the product and changed its research and development efforts.

There was considerable agreement that although genetic testing would grow progressively more important over the next decade or so, the largest market for DNA testing would always be in infectious diseases. Cancer testing, tissue typing, and personal identification (parentage, forensics) were also expected to continue to command a larger market than genetic testing. A number of respondents said that growth in genetic testing had been slower than they had anticipated in the late 1980s.

How companies answered our questions about expected growth seemed to be related to their situation in the market. Thus, to a large corporation developing testing technology the market has not "grown much at all." All that is underway is "specialty testing" and the "big players" in diagnostics "have not gotten into it."(v, 13)[j] In contrast, to a small company aiming to market more "esoteric" tests to a medical specialty such as oncology or neurology, the market already looks significant and poised for further expansion.

One small startup technology development company, founded in the late 1980s, originally expected its business to center around genetic testing. It ended up shifting to other applications, such as parentage in both humans and purebred animals, because raising money to develop genetic tests was too difficult. Investor confidence was reduced by regulatory uncertainties, the absence of a "well worn path to commercialization," and the realization that testing for single gene disorders, such as CF, that many had initially expected to be easy, turned out to be hard.

The commercial sector is not suffering because of competition from testing in academic centers, although genetic and cytogenetic testing were, for many years, largely in their province. Several company respondents reported that many medical school labs that perform genetic tests are losing money and require subsidies from their respective universities. This was consistent with the statements of the directors of university-based labs we visited, who all reported that their labs did not break even on genetic tests. The small scale of genetic testing sometimes made it difficult for them to get additional resources from the large parent laboratories at the medical centers.

Factors Affecting Growth of Genetic Testing

Technological Immaturity. Both the providers of testing services and the companies developing testing technologies saw the development of cheap, high-throughput testing systems as critically important to DNA testing in general and to genetic testing in particular. Many people's "wish lists" seemed to feature technological platforms that would allow one to test for large numbers of mutations at a reasonable cost. One scientist, active in test development, argued that the lack of such systems was a major reason that genetic testing remained an "expensive" and "underutilized" technology.

> If there are 400 different mutations in the gene, ... [that disease is] not amenable to...very inexpensive techniques.... Those techniques, on the other hand, that give you all of the information that a gene contains—sequencing at the ultimate extreme—are intrinsically low throughput, costly, and time-consuming. That's the dilemma.... The techniques that give you all the information are not suited for the clinical laboratory, either in terms of format, cost, throughput, turnaround time. Those that have more the feel of a clinical laboratory test in terms of turnaround time, throughput and cost,

---

[j]The Roman numeral refers to the organization; the Arabic number refers to the transcript page where the relevant discussion begins.

don't give you all the information you want and sometimes don't even give you enough information. (iv, 19)

A multinational company, successfully selling DNA-based tests for several infectious diseases in the United States, had developed a prototype test kit for a single-gene disorder and had placed the kit into a clinical trial in Europe with the goal of eventually marketing it to clinical laboratories as a replacement to home brew tests in the U.S. However, the European laboratories preferred their own home brews over the company's standardized product because they could flexibly adapt their home brew tests to the mutations prevalent in their respective countries. Accordingly, the company shifted the project back into the research phase, with the goal of eventually offering a test, perhaps based on a new testing technology, that would cover a much larger number of mutations.

Because of rapid change, companies that were primarily offering services did not want to invest a lot in new technologies. Companies were more interested in acquiring new test technologies from academe and altering them to get the test to perform in a reliable and cost-effective way at higher volume. An official at one large clinical lab explained:

> We made the decision that we could not invent the tests and so we went to established academic centers in which the tests were up and running, validated against clinical specimens and had a track record, and we negotiated licensing agreements to basically buy the technology. When we got it, we made some changes to make it work better in our hands, to satisfy ourselves that it behaved the way we thought it should...(i, 8)

Clinical Considerations. Genetic tests for inherited disease and predispositions need only be conducted once per patient, placing an upper limit on the market size, whereas people are tested repeatedly throughout their lifetimes for infectious diseases. Similarly, in the oncology context, many envision the use of DNA testing for ongoing monitoring of cancer patients, which would require running repeated assays. For this reason, some firms involved in DNA testing were devoting few resources to genetic testing.

A recurrent theme was the problem of test sensitivity, the ability of the test to detect all disease-causing mutations. A company offering genetic testing services, said:

> It's rarely just one mutation equals one genetic problem. So the problem [is] having really good screening tests. And what makes a good screening test? Are you happy with 70 percent [sensitivity]? Does it need to be 85 to 90 percent accurate? ...CF is pretty good. I mean, 70 percent with one [mutation] and...[with] a panel of up to 20 more you can get 85 percent. But you are never going to get 100 percent... Then we went into fragile X and triple repeats because that essentially is something [where]...one test is going to give you your answer....There really weren't a lot of genetic diseases that we could screen cost effectively and produce effectively, just because there's so many mutations that are involved. (x, 7)

Clinical utility is not always evident in testing for inherited disorders for which treatments have not yet been developed.

> If you are diagnosing something in human genetics that there's no treatment for, and no one's quite sure what the outcome is because you're looking at predisposition to disease, no one's going to buy your test. (ii, 10)

Financial Considerations. Because most single-gene disorders are rare, the demand for some genetic tests is likely to be very low. One provider of testing services commented that some of these tests were

> very low volume tests. You'd get one a year or one a month to do. So from a business perspective it was not cost effective to do, and you just have to drop it. (viii, 9)

Another way of attempting to deal with low volume tests for rare diseases is to send them out to "boutique" labs. But this is not profitable; by law, the sending lab can only charge what it is charged plus a small handling fee. The alternative, establishing a new test in house is also costly, so the company needs to determine: "Do we lose more setting it up or sending it out?" (xi, 8)

High costs also reduce demand. One provider of genetic testing services noted:

> Patients don't want to pay $200 or $600 for a genetic test. So we want to find technology platforms that allow us to drive the costs down so that maybe we're talking $35, $50 for a test rather than several hundred. So we've got to be making investments in technology platforms and looking for ways to streamline processes. (i, 15)

The director of one university laboratory pointed out that the costs of clinical testing go far beyond the technology itself.

> Somebody [has] to review the results and interpret the results and issue the reports, and all the phone calls back and forth, and stuff like that... It's just my feeling from personal experience that those are a significant part of our total cost.(xiv,33)

A number of companies consider reimbursement when they decide to develop a new test. One provider of services said,

> If the test is going to cost us $1,000 and we get so few referrals we have to do them one at a time, and we're only going to get reimbursed $200, then I'm not going to do it.(xv, 10)

Another commented:

> We have a lot of sales reps out in the field talking to physicians and oncologists who say, "you know it would be nice if we had such and such a test." Eventually all of that filters back and we make some effort into investigating would it be possible for us to do. Would it fit? Is there a market? Is there a reimbursement for it? Is it potentially going to wind up making money? And then [we] go ahead and try and make a deal, bring the technology, offer it. (vii, 8)

In considering whether to offer a particular test, some respondents said they would consider how it fit with their existing offerings. A low volume test might be added even if it was not cost effective by itself if it "completed an offering" in a particular clinical area.

> If you could offer the whole gamut [of tests for a number of related diseases] there might be a value, an added value to the [physician],...because he is going down the differential [diagnosis]....So it's not just numbers driven; it's also how it completes sort of a profile or presentation.(ix, 16)

Ethical Considerations. The controversial nature of testing for inherited disease or predispositions, and the ethical questions raised by predictive genetic testing, also seemed to discourage a focus on this area. One company with a generic technology hesitated to enter the genetic testing arena.

> I mean, the minute you go into human inherited disease and predisposition, then there's ethical issues. So what we did is look at the three market segments--inherited disease, cancer, and infectious disease--and said from a business point of view, what are the largest markets today? Basically almost all the pie is in infectious disease....And there's no ethical issues and you're replacing the initial products by bringing in something that is easier to use and cheaper and is just better for the health care system. So our primary market focus is on infectious disease for that very reason. (iii,5)

A biotechnology startup company founded in the late 1980s, was more specific. This company had developed technology for detecting mutations that it expected to apply to some of the more common Mendelian diseases, such as cystic fibrosis and neurofibromatosis.

> CF was going to be a very large focus for the company....The management and the board...were for a time much more interested when they thought that population screening was going to be a reality. Now I guess our opinion is that it won't be ever, so that means the market is much smaller. (vii, 8)

Like the other startup discussed above, this company has redirected its efforts, in this case toward somatic cell testing and gene therapy.

<u>Regulatory Considerations.</u> Regulatory issues loom large, particularly to small startups interested in developing kits or reagents that clinical labs could use to perform tests. Regulatory uncertainty in the case of genetic tests stemmed in part from the novelty of the tests. One small test technology developer told us:

> In genetic diagnostics there never was a reliable test for a lot of those diseases....So you could never test for those things before. So no one was clear on how it would ever be regulated and what level of sensitivity you would need.(ii, 9)

The company thus shifted its strategy away from genetic testing, placing highest priority on parentage testing, followed by infectious disease, cancer, and genetic testing in that order.

Another technology development company was using its technology to test livestock for inherited susceptibility to disease—an application it chose in part because it is at present unregulated by government agencies (vi).

One technology development company experienced longer regulatory delays than it had previously when it sought FDA approval for an infectious disease test using new DNA technology. Despite evidence provided by the company, FDA was skeptical that the sensitivity of the test, which had previously been used exclusively in research, was as good a clinical test as the company maintained.

Laboratory Quality Assurance

All of the test providers seemed confident that their own efforts to maintain quality were effective, appropriate, and in compliance with the relevant laws. Several respondents said they believed that most laboratories did good work, but also suggested that laboratory quality was uneven and that some companies and medical center laboratories were not performing adequate work. One official at a technology development company who had been active in a proficiency testing program said:

> We had a couple of places that really didn't do all that well [in proficiency tests]. They shouldn't have been testing for certain things that they were. Some of these people were people who now have the diploma -- they're clinical molecular geneticists -- but in the proficiency testing they didn't score all that well....A lot of places are good, but some places are not so good. All of them give diagnoses. [laughs] (f, 37)[k]

Another respondent stated that he had seen poor results used to make important decisions and argued that physicians often had little choice but to rely on word-of-mouth assessments of laboratory quality:

> "Well, did you send it to such and such a laboratory?" "No, we sent it over there." "Well, you know so and so's laboratory is a better shop." And I think that that's the way, I think that's the status of genetic testing in the United

---

[k] From this point, lower case letters refer to the respondent. This new code is intended to help preserve the anonymity of responding organizations.

States right now. There are some laboratories that are considered very good and there are some that are considered not so good. (g, 14ff)

As the above discussion suggests, there were differences in attitudes about the extent to which uneven laboratory quality was a serious problem.

Most providers of testing services were wary of additional FDA involvement in regulating home brew testing. According to some respondents, regulation of home brew testing would reduce the availability of testing for rare diseases, would slow innovation, and would lead tests to be underutilized. Several respondents argued that the procedures in place at most clinical laboratories for maintaining quality were by and large adequate and that regulation "would delay work and would cost a lot of money and really wouldn't do that much for quality." (b, 37)

Institutional Review Boards (IRBs)

IRB review occurred at a variety of organizations, including companies that provide testing services, technology development companies, and medical center laboratories. At the companies, officials typically said that they relied on the IRBs of collaborating universities to review their research protocols. One company, however, described how it had established its own IRB using external advisors to provide review of its protocols for conducting studies of the validity of tests.

Companies that acquire the rights to tests developed and validated elsewhere, and who then modify the protocols to make them work in their hands or on a large scale, often do not classify this as research which would be subject to IRB review. However, respondents described several other forms of internal review. Some of the largest organizations had formal procedures or committees for reviewing new test protocols to determine if they were ready to be offered as a clinical service. At some smaller organizations, the senior personnel collectively or, in some cases individually, made such assessments.

The Gatekeeping Function of Laboratories

Interviewees agreed that genetic counseling and informed consent were essential aspects of medical genetics, but they disagreed about the role of the testing laboratory in performing and verifying that counseling and consent had occurred. One source of the differences in opinion seemed to be the different professional practices that have evolved in the fields of laboratory medicine and pathology, on the one hand, and human genetics, on the other. The director of a medical center clinical laboratory who had a laboratory medicine orientation explained that his laboratory's "relationship is with the physician, or whoever is ordering the test" and that "the question of obtaining informed consent for testing is the responsibility of the person who orders the test and sees the patient."(b,31)

In contrast, the director of another medical center laboratory who had a human genetics orientation, suggested that laboratory medicine and pathology should (and perhaps are beginning to) shift more toward the approach of geneticists. The main differences in orientation, she argued, concerned counseling and informed consent, for which the geneticists believed that the lab should take a more active role.

I think that, you know, testing labs have somewhat of a responsibility to track down and try to get the referrals done appropriately for the benefit of the family. For example, did [the family] know the implications of [the

110

test], that if the child turns out to be positive, they won't get disability insurance or life insurance and will be marked for many years to come and all those implications....I think it's really important that the family be steered into genetic counseling and that the referring physician is educated in some way that there are other critical factors than just sending the blood to the lab and getting an answer back. (h, 9)

Differences of opinion on this matter were also found among commercial clinical laboratories. One official explained:

For all of our tests we have policies about who will consent to tests.... And on top of that we are laying on a required informed consent that the patient has to fill out with their physician so that they know what we are about. (e, 17ff)

Another company had developed ethical guidelines:

For accepting samples...we won't do testing if we know...that it's just for sex selection....The same can be true for testing minors, [and] testing individuals who are at risk for different diseases that may not have had informed consent. (i, 30)

In contrast, several other biotechnology companies argued that the role of the laboratory should be limited to assuring the reliability of the results it reports.

I've thought a lot about this, that the way to think about this is about physician autonomy. A physician wants a piece of information to judge his patient on. What the labs ought to be required to do is to make sure that they provide the physician with the information that the physician...asked for....The lab ought not to be in the business of practicing medicine. (j, 23)

An official at another company contended that there was insufficient justification for treating DNA tests differently, and that to require laboratories to act as gatekeepers represents "an inappropriate placement of the gate" (k, 26ff).

Some providers of testing services employed genetic counselors and some did not. Officials at a testing company that did not, and which serves a national market, argued genetic counseling is part of "hands-on patient care," not laboratory work, and that it therefore should be part of the local care that is offered to the patient by the physician. This company always provided physicians who ordered tests with a thorough interpretation of the result (c, 43). Another company, one of the largest players in the national clinical laboratory market, operated a counseling unit that included two genetic counselors and a number of less highly trained "case managers." This firm required use of its own consent form for some but not all genetic tests (a, 7ff).

Closely related to the question of the extent to which genetic testing laboratories should serve as gatekeepers was the question of the extent to which regulatory authorities or professional groups should be able to restrict the tests available to individual patients. An official at a large clinical laboratory argued:

I don't think a regulator should determine that a patient, if they're educated, should or shouldn't get tested. I think that should be the patient and the patient's family decision of whether to get tested, but not without education. I'm not saying anybody should be able to walk in and just say "I want it 'cause I want it." I think we do have an obligation to make sure they understand the test, what its limitations are and understand what a positive and a negative will each mean, but if they, after that kind of understanding, request that the test still be done, I think that should be their decision. (a, 12)

Interpretation of Test Results

Many respondents who provide testing services said that an important aspect of their work was giving physicians the information they need to understand the meaning of tests and interpret results properly. These educational efforts were needed, according to most respondents, because genetic testing represents a new area to most practicing physicians. At the large testing companies, the task of educating physicians entailed not only providing detailed reports on the meaning of each patient's results, but also producing and distributing a variety of educational materials for physicians. (Editor's note: See Appendix 4, Cho *et al*: Analysis of Informational Materials About Genetic Tests.) As one official put it: "[For] a lot of physicians...this is really a very, very new area and they really need our help and will probably always need our help." (a, 8)

Another test provider argued that changes in the health care system were making it increasingly important for test providers to help physicians understand tests:

> More and more front line medicine is done by family and general providers rather than subspecialists. So we have. . .to make sure that the clients can get the information they need quickly when they call about what the test means, what tests need to be done, what other samples do they need. (c, 29)

Testing of Minors

The testing of minors for adult-onset disorders or carrier status was a matter about which there was some divergence of views. Some companies fully supported prohibitions on testing of minors for adult-onset disease or carrier status. In contrast, one company official argued that he did not believe that companies necessarily should be involved in deciding such matters as testing of minors. This company had nonetheless made a commitment to follow the consensus of the genetics community. A third perspective held that the question of whether testing of minors was appropriate required a case by case, disease by disease assessment by an experienced physician, suggesting that any guidelines he would support have to allow for considerable professional discretion. For example, one argued that in the case of familial polyposis knowing the test result might greatly benefit a child by eliminating the need for repeated colonoscopies. In other cases, where the test outcome would not have immediate clinical implications, testing might not be warranted until the age of majority.

Patents and Royalties

One policy area that respondents themselves repeatedly brought up was the question of the proper uses of intellectual property in genetic testing. In particular, a number of organizations, both companies and medical center laboratories, expressed concern that intellectual property policies would drive up the price of tests or otherwise adversely affect test availability. Several respondents worried that when patent holders grant companies exclusive licenses to genetic tests, this could limit access to necessary testing by limiting the number of laboratories and increasing the price. Respondents argued that the granting of numerous patents, each on a specific mutation in the same gene, could make testing unaffordable if each patent holder demanded a royalty. For example, an official at one testing company suggested that university technology transfer offices were filing large numbers of patents, with the result that providers of any effective genetic test might need to pay multiple, or "stacked" royalties, producing "a diagnostic test that no one can afford." (d, 40)

DISCUSSION

In a survey conducted by one of us in 1986 only 118 biotechnology companies could be identified who were likely to be engaged in genetic testing, and of the 85 companies that replied, only 22 said they were developing or offering tests for genetic or chromosome disorders.[1] In this survey, conducted ten years later, we identified five times as many companies likely to be involved in genetic testing. Among respondents, 6.7 times as many companies as in 1986—147 firms—were engaged in genetic testing activity. Clearly commercial interest has grown.

In 1986, it was virtually impossible to perform genetic tests for common, complex disorders. Although such testing is now possible only for a handful of disorders, it is genetic testing for the common disorders that has sparked the most commercial interest. Respondents to the earlier survey indicated that the disease characteristic of greatest importance in genetic test development was prevalence of the disease. The data ten years later (Table 3) bears this out. Although a few companies have developed tests for rare diseases, this has been mostly to gain a foothold in the field or to provide a complete battery of testing for the specialties on which they concentrate.

Despite this dramatic increase in activity, the field is far from maturity. Many more companies are engaged in research and development of genetic tests than are delivering genetic test kits or services (Table 2). Several companies perceive the market growing at a slower rate than they anticipated in the 1980s.

Scientific, clinical, technological, and ethical factors are all at work. Many diseases, including common complex ones such as breast and colon cancer, occur in the presence of any one of hundreds of different inherited mutations, or in the absence of any of them. Moreover, some people who have inherited mutations that contribute to disease occurrence in others will never get the disease over a normal lifetime. Current technology for providing tests for disorders in which multiple mutations contribute to disease causation is expensive and ponderous. Given these limitations, tests for common disorders will attract greater interest than tests for rare disorders. Several interviewees pointed to the precarious financial rewards of testing for rare diseases; they need tests for which the demand is likely to be high. This is much more probable for common disorders, even if the tests are imperfect. Further, unless they hold the patents for the key materials or processes, companies may be limited in testing or may also have to pay licensing fees on materials or processes to the patent holders. Several interviewees complained about the high costs of licensing, and a recent effort to collect royalties on the use of a patented reagent in prenatal screening bears this out.[2]

Recent advances, particularly employing chip technology,[3] bode well for much simpler and less expensive technology that will be capable of detecting hundreds if not thousands of different mutations simultaneously. The ability to detect protein gene products of disease-related genes may also provide a more sensitive and more functional test than direct searching for mutations at the DNA level.[4]

From our interviews, we suspect that potential test developers are awaiting the arrival of faster throughput, less expensive, and more sensitive technologies that have a greater chance of being reimbursed by health insurers. Even then, the less-than-perfect predictability of genetic tests for several disorders, as well as the absence of interventions of proven effectiveness for many inherited diseases, may deter their entrance into the field.

Those engaged in genetic testing told us that ethical issues were a consideration. These included not only controversy over genetic testing but the role of the laboratory in assuring that patients were adequately informed of and consented to the test, and the testing of minors. Interviewees differed on how much responsibility the clinical laboratory had and how much belonged to physicians ordering tests. Concerns over ethical issues has probably contributed to relatively few organizations marketing directly to patients and other consumers, although a few do.

Many companies see other uses of recombinant DNA technology, particularly for diagnosis of infectious diseases, as a more certain market. Only 16 companies were devoting more than 10 percent of their resources to activities related to genetic testing.

The state of the technology has, in part, dictated the activities of genetic testing companies. Except when it is sufficient to test for a small number of mutations, current technology does not permit the tests to be assembled in kits and marketed to clinical laboratories. Consequently, biotechnology companies have gone into the clinical laboratory business themselves, marketing genetic testing *services* rather than *kits*. This has also proved to be less of a regulatory hurdle because FDA, although having the authority to regulate new testing services, has elected not to. One biotechnology company that is offering genetic testing states in its prospectus for common stock that "the company's genetic testing laboratory is regulated under CLIA, which imposes less complex regulatory guidelines than those required by the FDA."[1,5]

The question arises of whether tests currently being developed and marketed have been subject to adequate external review. Under CLIA, clinical laboratories must show the analytic validity and reliability of the tests they perform, but not their clinical validity or utility. We were interested, therefore, in other means by which developers of test services subject new tests to review. This is all the more important for tests developed in-house (home brews) which are subject to no external review other than under CLIA. Approximately half of the BTCs and NPOs who offered genetic testing services reported using home brews. Although over 80 percent of commercial and university-based laboratories that were offering genetic services said their tests were assessed before being made available routinely, two mechanisms that might suggest formal review—submission to an IRB and communication with FDA—were not used by nearly that many. IRBs do not review data on test validity and utility, but submission of a protocol to an IRB indicates that the organization is systematically collecting data. Moreover, under regulations pursuant to the Medical Device Amendments to the Food, Drug and Cosmetic Act, organizations attempting to establish the clinical

---

[1] Over two-thirds of respondents agreed that current FDA policies, or lack of FDA policies, hindered the development of safe and effective genetic tests. Unfortunately, the statement did not distinguish between the two possibilities. (Table 5)

validity of an *in vitro* diagnostic device, such as a genetic test kit or specific probe, must operate under a protocol approved by an IRB and, when there is no independent means of confirming the test, must obtain an Investigational Device Exemption (IDE) from FDA. Only two respondents had obtained IDEs. The low use of IDEs probably reflects the intention of test developers to market their tests as services, which, as we have mentioned, FDA has elected not to regulate. If FDA were to regulate new devices whose developer intend to market them as services, they would probably not be deluged with applications, considering the relatively low rate of commercial development of genetic tests.

Once tests are marketed, they are subject to CLIA regulations. As CLIA does not have separate requirements for laboratories offering DNA-based genetic testing, a laboratory need only demonstrate general, good laboratory practices. Voluntary proficiency testing programs were available at the time of the survey, and informal sharing of unknown specimens to compare results is a longstanding clinical laboratory practice. Nevertheless, 11.1 percent of BTCs offering genetic testing services and 16.5 percent of NPO molecular laboratories did not participate in either formal or informal proficiency testing programs. In the interviews, several commercial laboratory directors told us they were aware of poor quality laboratories who were offering services. They pointed out that information on the quality of laboratories spreads by word of mouth. There is no systematic method of informing providers and patients of laboratories that have demonstrated high quality performance.

SUMMARY AND CONCLUSIONS

Compared to a decade ago, genetic testing activity has grown among both commercial biotechnology companies (BTC) and nonprofit organizations (NPOs). Growth has been in generic testing technologies, development of tests for specific diseases, and provision of testing services. Many BTCs engaged in genetic testing, and a smaller proportion of NPOs are developing or offering tests for common complex disorders.

Growth is slower than many observers anticipated for a variety of interconnected reasons. Current test technologies have limited clinical sensitivity, technology is expected to change, the market is limited because it is only necessary to test a person once for a given genetic condition, the clinical utility of some tests is questionable and that makes demand uncertain, many genetic disorders occur at a low frequency, tests sometimes pose ethical and financial considerations, and regulations are still uncertain.

Technology development companies and large clinical multipurpose clinical laboratories do not view the market for genetic testing as particularly profitable in the short term. It is not clear how rapidly they will develop and market new tests for either common or rare disorders. At the same time, one cannot conclude that these companies will not move forward on genetic testing in the long run. In particular, new technologies for rapid and low-cost genotyping, which are being demonstrated in infectious diseases and somatic cell testing, might readily spread to germline diagnostics, particularly when they provide clinical data useful enough to warrant the testing.

Tests under development often do not receive external review. Several BTCs and NPOs that are developing genetic tests, including tests for complex disorders, and some organizations using home brews in offering testing services, fail to make use of institutional review boards (IRBs), obtain investigational device exemptions from the Food and Drug Administration (FDA), or submit the tests to FDA review.

Quality assurance of laboratories offering genetic tests is uneven. Most laboratories offering molecular genetic tests are registered under the Clinical Laboratory Improvement Amendments (CLIA), but participation in proficiency testing programs for genetic tests is not required of CLIA-certified laboratories. Eleven percent of NBTCs and 16 percent of NPO molecular laboratories did not participate in either formal or informal proficiency testing programs.

Commercial laboratory directors told us that they were aware of poor quality laboratories who were offering services. They pointed out that information on the quality of laboratories spreads via word of mouth and that there is no systematic way for health care providers or patients to identify laboratories that have demonstrated high quality performance. These findings raise questions as to whether current policies assure the quality of laboratories offering genetic testing.

Both BTCs and NPOs are marketing to nongeneticist physicians. Education of physicians in the proper interpretation of genetic tests poses an ongoing challenge. The majority of respondents from both BTCs and NPOs disagree with the statement that "most physicians can interpret genetic tests adequately to the patients".

Those interviewed disagreed considerably concerning the extent to which the testing laboratories should insist on compliance with ethical and clinical guidelines, especially regarding informed consent and the indications for testing. Overall, the study suggests that patients and test providers would both benefit from clarification of policies.

ABOUT THE AUTHORS

Neil (Tony) Holtzman is Professor of Pediatrics at the Johns Hopkins University School of Medicine. He holds joint appointments in Health Policy and Epidemiology at The Johns Hopkins School of Hygiene and Public Health. Holtzman is also director of Genetics and Public Policy Studies at The Johns Hopkins Medical Institutions. He is Acting Chair of the Maryland Advisory Council on Hereditary and Congenital Disorders and was a member of the NIH-DOE Working Group on Ethical, Legal, and Social Implications of Human Genome Research while it was extant. He was Chair of the Working Group's Task Force on Genetic Testing.

Stephen Hilgartner is Assistant Professor in the Department of Science and Technology Studies at Cornell University. He specializes in social studies of contemporary biology, biotechnology, and medicine. Currently, his main research project is an extended ethnographic study of the social world of genome mapping and sequencing.

REFERENCES

1. N. A. Holtzman. *Proceed with Caution: Predicting Genetic Risks in the Recombinant DNA Era*. Chapter 6 (Baltimore: Johns Hopkins: 1989).

2. K. Eichenwald. Push for royalties threatens use of down syndrome test. *New York Times* p. 1. May 23, 1977.

3. J. G. Hacia, L. C. Brody, M. S. Chee, S. P. Fodor and F. S. Collins. Detection of heterozygous mutations in BRCA1 using high density oligonucleotide arrays and two-colour fluorescence analysis. *Nature Genetics* 14:441-447 (1996).

4. M. A. Telatar, Z. Wang, N. Udar, et al. Ataxia-telangiectasia: mutations in ATM cDNA detected by protein-truncation sequencing. *Am J Hum Genet* 59:40-44 (1996).

5. Myriad Genetics, Inc Prospectus. 2,600,000 Shares. Myriad Genetics, Inc. Common Stock. Salt Lake City: Myriad Genetics, Inc. Cowen & Co., USB Securities, Inc. October 5, 1995.

TABLE 1

CATEGORIES COVERED IN THE QUESTIONNAIRE

Genetic testing activities (basic research; development of genetic test services, kits, or other products; offering of testing services or kits)

Patenting and licensing (patents applied for or issued, licensing agreements)

Specific diseases (44 conditions listed plus opportunity to write in; for each: development stage, target group, intended use, test methodology)

Marketing practices or plans (marketing targets, informational material, and distribution methods)

Support for development of tests

Financial issues [for companies only] (percent of resources for genetic testing activities, current and estimated future revenues from testing)

Assessment of genetic testing technologies

Regulatory issues (use of Institutional Review Boards (IRBs), contacts with Food and Drug Administration, registered under Clinical Laboratory Improvement Amendments (CLIA)

Personal opinions (FDA, CLIA, laboratory quality, physicians knowledge, privacy of genetic information)

Genetic test interpretations and counseling activities (employment of a counselor, communication of results, testing of minors)

Clinical laboratory issues (quality control, use of home brews, participation in proficiency testing)

TABLE 2

EXTENT AND TYPE OF GENETIC TESTING ACTIVITY

	BTCs[a]		NPOs[b]	
	n	**(%)**	**n**	**(%)**
Engaged in any test-related activity (TOTAL)	147	(31.9)	316	(89.5)
Developing genetic tests (not marketing)	20	(13.6)	1	(.3)
Services [c]	7		1	
Kits [c]	18		0	
Currently marketing genetic tests (not developing)	12	(8.2)	124	(39.2)
Services	11		124	
Kits 1		0		
Both developing and currently marketing	26	(17.7)	160	(50.6)
Services [c]	18		160	
Kits [c]	9		3	
Other (Primarily research and ancillary products)	89	(60.5)	31	(9.8)

[a] Biotechnology companies
[b] Nonprofit organizations
[c] Numbers on these two rows can be greater than the totals on the preceding row because the same organization may be developing or marketing services and kits.

TABLE 3

ORGANIZATIONS ENGAGED IN GENETIC TESTING FOR CERTAIN DISORDERS

| Disorders | Developing or Providing Tests | | | |
| | BTCs | | NPOs | |
	n	(%)[c]	n	(%)[c]
Any of 44	53	(100.0)	212	(100.0)
3 Complex [a] (not 3 single-gene)	18	(34.0)	9	(4.2)
3 Single-gene [b] (not 3 complex)	9	(17.0)	99	(46.7)
Both	16	(30.2)	38	(17.9)
Neither	10	(18.8)	66	(31.2)

X^2 p<0.0001

[a] Complex = Alzheimer's, breast cancer, colon cancer (HNPCC)
[b] Single-gene = cystic fibrosis, fragile X, muscular dystrophy
[c] % of all organizations engaged in testing for any of 44 disorders

TABLE 4

SUBMISSION OF GENETIC TEST PROTOCOLS TO INSTITUTIONAL REVIEW BOARDS (IRBs) OR CONTACT WITH THE FOOD AND DRUG ADMINISTRATION (FDA) REGARDING GENETIC TESTING

	BTCs		NPOs	
	n	(%)	n	(%)
Developing genetic tests (not offering) (TOTAL)	15	(100.0)	1	(100.0)
Ever submitted to an IRB (not FDA)	7	(46.7)	1	(100.0)
Ever contacted FDA (not IRB)	0	0	0	0
Submitted to an IRB and contacted FDA	2	(13.3)	0	0
Currently offering genetic tests (not developing)(TOTAL)	6	(100.0)	88	(100.0)
Ever submitted to an IRB (not FDA)	2	(33.3)	34	(38.6)
Ever contacted FDA (not IRB)	0	0	2	(2.3)
Submitted to an IRB and contacted FDA	0	0	1	(1.1)
Both developing and currently offering (TOTAL)	22	(100.0)	12	(100.0)
Ever submitted to an IRB (not FDA)	5	(22.7)	126	(65.1)
Ever contacted FDA (not IRB)	2	(9.1)	82	0
Submitted to an IRB and contacted FDA	9	(40.9)	0	(11.1)
			14	
Homebrews (TOTAL)	14	(100.0)	95	(100.0)
Ever submitted to an IRB (not FDA)	2	(14.3)	63	(66.3)
Ever contacted FDA (not IRB)	2	(14.3)	0	0
Submitted to an IRB and contacted FDA	6	(42.9)	9	(9.5)

TABLE 5

QUALITY ASSURANCE ACTIVITIES AMONG ORGANIZATIONS OFFERING GENETIC TEST SERVICES

| | | | NPOs | | | |
| | BTCs | | Molecular | | Cytogenetic | |
	n	(%) yes	n	(%) yes	n	(%) yes
CLIA						
Total answering question	27	(100.0)	97	(100.0)	86	(100.0)
Registered under CLIA [a]	23	(85.2)	84	(86.6)	86	(100.0)
Proficiency Testing (PT)						
Total answering question	27	(100.0)	93	(100.0)	89	(100.0)
Participate in formal PT	12	(44.4)	37	(37.4)	56	(62.9)
Share unknowns informally	3	(11.1)	11	(11.1)	1	(1.1)
Both	9	(33.3)	35	(35.4)	32	(36.0)
Neither	3	(11.1)	16	(16.5)	0	0

[a] Clinical Laboratory Improvement Amendment 1988

122

TABLE 6

MARKETING TARGETS FOR LABORATORIES CURRENTLY OFFERING GENETIC TESTING SERVICES

Target Group	BTCs		NPOs Molecular		NPOs Cytogenetic	
	n	(%)	n	(%)	n	(%)
Total answering question	25	(100.0)	117	(100.0)	105	(100.0)
Geneticist/genetic counselors	21	(84.0)	99	(84.6)	78	(74.3)
Non-genetics specialists	23	(92.0)	98	(83.8)	95	(90.5)
Managed care organizations	20	(80.0)	51	(43.6)	54	(51.45) p<.005[a]
Primary care physicians	17	(68.0)	74	(63.2)	76	(72.4)
Patients/consumers	7	(28.0)	45	(38.5)	49	(46.7)

[a] X^2 between BTCs and NPOs

TABLE 7

PERSONAL AGREEMENT WITH STATEMENTS ON GENETIC TESTING[a]

| Statement | Respondents Agreeing | | | | |
| | BTCs (N=81) | | NPOs (N=245) | | |
	n (%)	mean (+ sd)	n (%)	mean (+sd)	p (t-test)
"Most physicians can interpret genetic test results adequately to their patients."	16 (20)	3.1 (.72)	14 (6)	3.6 (.63)	<.001
"Current policies under the Clinical Laboratory Improvement Act assure the quality of genetic test services."	38 (53)	2.5 (.75)	89 (39)	2.8 (.84)	=0.01
"An industry-wide ethical code for test development and marketing would improve the quality of genetic test services."	68 (84)	1.9 (.71)	204 (85)	1.8 (.79)	NS
"Current FDA policies, or lack of policies, hinder the development of safe and effective genetic test kits or other products."	52 (67)	2.1 (.95)	165 (75)	2.0 (.83)	NS
"Some laboratories that offer genetic testing lack adequate quality assurance programs."	62 (85)	1.9 (.67)	197 (84)	1.8 (.75)	NS
"Additional laws or regulations are needed to ensure the privacy of genetic information."	51 (67)	2.1 (1.0)	177 (74)	2.0 (.89)	NS

[a] Scale: 1 = agree strongly; 2 = agree somewhat; 3 = disagree somewhat; 4 = disagree strongly

APPENDIX 4. INFORMATIONAL MATERIALS ABOUT GENETIC TESTS[a]

M. K. Cho[b,c] Ph.D.; M. Arruda,[b] N. A. Holtzman,[d] M.D., M.P.H.

INTRODUCTION

As genetic testing moves into the mainstream of health care in the United States, patients and providers will have more need for basic test information. We surveyed informational materials available in 1995 and summarize our results here. In general, the materials tended to contain information that would aid in determining a patient's eligibility for a genetic test, but lacked sufficient information about the tests themselves, such as their sensitivity, specificity or predictive value, the purpose of testing, and information concerning patient rights.

The increasing need for genetic testing information is stimulated by two main factors. First, the number of genetic tests ordered is increasing, in part because tests to predict genetic risk of common conditions such as cardiovascular disease, Alzheimer disease, or breast cancer are now available.

Second, the resultant increasing demand for and volume of tests may not occur with a corresponding increase in availability of genetic counseling for patients or consultations between genetic specialists and nonspecialist health care providers.

Consequently, genetic tests will increasingly be administered by providers without genetic training. The lack of training and of educational materials might already have contributed to providers' and patients' misunderstanding of test results and implications. A recent study of colon cancer testing found that physicians who had ordered the test misinterpreted the results nearly a third of the time.[1]

Written educational materials can be used either with,[2] or instead of, other educational forms such as video.[3] Evidence shows that many patients prefer written materials, that they are effective for communicating medical information[4] and that materials such as booklets effectively decrease anxiety about medical procedures.[5] Written materials are especially useful as an adjunct to counseling sessions.

Written informational materials have been specifically recommended for genetic test .[6] Use and interpretation of the tests is complex and testing can lead to social discrimination[7,8,9,10,11] and can have unanticipated psychological impact.[12,13,14,15,16,17] Indeed, several policymaking bodies have been concerned about the risks and potential for inappropriate use of genetic tests, so they specified the key types of content that should be provided to patients if they are to make informed choices about testing.[18,19,20,21]

---

[a]This paper was requested by the Chair of the Task Force. It is an extension of the survey of biotechnology companies and nonprofit clinical laboratories described in Appendix 3. The views expressed in this paper are those of the authors and do not necessarily reflect the views of the Task Force.
[b]Center for Bioethics University of Pennsylvania, Philadelphia, PA
[c]Department of Molecular and Cellular Engineering, University of Pennsylvania, Philadelphia, PA
[d]Genetics and Public Policy Studies, Johns Hopkins Medical Institutions, Baltimore, MD

We surveyed the extent to which existing informational materials on genetic tests contain key elements that are necessary if patients and providers are to evaluate the purpose, accuracy, risks, and benefits of that test.[22] Further, we analyzed whether for-profit and nonprofit organizations differed in the inclusion of particular key elements.

METHODS

Identification of Organizations Providing Informational Materials

From the survey conducted for the Task Force on Genetic Testing (see Appendix 3) in early 1995, we identified 178 organizations, including biotechnology companies, molecular genetics laboratories, and cytogenetic laboratories, who said they had printed or audiovisual information about the genetic testing services or products they offered.[23]

Telephone Survey

In a telephone survey, we contacted each of the 178 organizations to determine which of them provided printed or audiovisual information about genetic tests to providers, patients, or both. We then determined: (a) for whom the materials were intended, (b) the context in which information was disseminated (e.g., by request only or to providers or patients on mailing lists), (c) whether the information was accompanied by counseling, and (d) who developed the materials. The study was approved by the University of Pennsylvania Committee on Studies Involving Human Beings (Assurance #M1025). Written informed consent forms were waived.

The first set of calls to all 178 organizations was made between October 1 and November 28, 1995. We made up to three follow-up calls and made one written contact with a letter and questionnaire to each organization, continuing through March 1996. We interviewed the person in the organization who would be most knowledgeable about the development and distribution of informational materials for our telephone survey.

From the previous mailed questionnaire, (see Appendix 3) we also had data on whether the organization was for-profit (e.g., biotechnology companies) or nonprofit (e.g., cytogenetics or molecular genetics laboratories at universities).

Collection and Content Analysis of Informational Materials

We requested copies of printed or audiovisual informational materials from all organizations that indicated that they provided such material. We chose material for content analysis if it concerned either diagnostic or predictive DNA-based genetic tests. The selected tests included those to detect hereditary disorders such as Duchenne muscular dystrophy, as well as those to detect chromosome abnormalities in tumors, such as specific translocations. We excluded material if it concerned tests that were not DNA-based (e.g., a test that detected blood lipid levels) or tests not for use on human samples. We also excluded materials that involved only tests used in newborn screening or involved only amniocentesis, chorionic villus sampling, and/or triple tests (for Down syndrome). These materials generally do not describe specific, individual tests, and thus were not comparable to the rest of the content analysis.

Virtually all the material we collected was in the form of printed pamphlets. We analyzed only the English versions, and merely recorded the availability of non-English versions. Some organizations provided general pamphlets (e.g., about the organization, about genetic testing or genetic inheritance generally, or about counseling) along with specific pamphlets about a test. In these cases, we considered the two pamphlets together as the unit of analysis, and will refer to them as "the pamphlet."

Using recommendations by several policy-making bodies about minimal elements of information that patients would need in order to assess a genetic test, we chose 10 elements and determined if they were present in the pamphlets (see Table 1).[24,25,26,27,28] A statement fitting any part of the description of each content element was counted as a presence of the element. For example, any mention of either sensitivity, specificity, predictive value, false positive or false negative rate of a test was counted as a statement on test performance. One member of the research team (M.A.) coded all of the materials, and another member (M.C.) independently analyzed a 20 percent subsample to determine the inter-rater reliability of the coding scheme. The percent agreement between raters for each element ranged from 88 percent to 96 percent, with an average agreement of 93 percent. The corresponding Kappa scores of inter-rater agreement ranged from 0.74 to 0.92. Because of the high level of agreement, we used only the data coded by M.A. for our analyses.

RESULTS

Some of the results of the content analysis were reported at the 1996 annual meeting of the American Society of Human Genetics[29] and a detailed report appears in the *American Journal of Medical Genetics.*[30] Those results are summarized briefly:

Ninety-five percent (169/178) of organizations responded to our survey; and 131/169 (78 percent) confirmed using informational materials. We analyzed 115 pamphlets collected from 125/131 (95 percent) of the organizations.

Overall, information about genetic testing was highly variable in content and potentially deficient or misleading. For example, nearly half of the pamphlets included some statement about the accuracy of the test, such as "more than 99 percent accurate" or "will detect all carriers," but most of these did not specify whether their statements referred to sensitivity, specificity, or predictive value.

The elements least frequently included in the pamphlets were risks and benefits, patient rights, and intended use or purpose of the test. Only 6.9 percent (2/29) of pamphlets intended for physicians, 26 percent (10/39) of those intended for patients, and 17 percent (8/47) intended for both included any explanation of risks and benefits of testing. Also, only 3.4 percent (1/29) of those intended for physicians, 26 percent (10/39) of those intended for patients, and 47 percent (22/47) of those intended for both mentioned confidentiality, voluntariness, or the possibility of discrimination in conjunction with genetic testing.

The most frequently included elements were descriptions of the conditions detected by the test (99/115; 86 percent), and the appropriate patients for testing (85/115; 74 percent).

Less than half of the materials included a statement on test performance (48/115; 42 percent). Approximately one in five pamphlets (24/115; 21 percent) included information on test interpretation.

<u>Content Elements by Profit Status of Organization</u>

In addition, we performed analyses to determine when key elements included in the materials were associated with the type of organization that developed the material (i.e., for-profit or nonprofit). Of the 115 pamphlets, 82 percent (94/115) came from nonprofit organizations, and 18 percent (21/115) came from for-profit organizations. The materials used by nonprofit organizations were more likely to be developed by or in conjunction with an external group such as the March of Dimes or Cystic Fibrosis Foundation (38/94; 40 percent) than the materials used by for-profit organizations (2/21; 9.5 percent) (P=0.02). Whereas most of the pamphlets developed by for-profit organizations were designed for use by both providers and patients (17/21; 81 percent), a substantial proportion of materials from nonprofits was intended for providers only (30/94; 32 percent).

We found that pamphlets from for-profit and nonprofit organizations did not differ significantly in whether they included seven of the ten key content elements listed in Table 1. A substantial proportion of material from both for-profit (11/21, 52 percent) and nonprofit organizations (30/94; 32 percent) consisted of a list of available tests accompanied by pamphlets that could be used in counseling. In many of these cases, the lists included price and shipping information (directed at providers), and the pamphlets tended to have information about diseases, rather than about the genetic tests for the diseases.

Only about one-fifth of the materials from either for-profit or nonprofit organizations had any statements on interpretation of test results.

When interpretation statements were included, they typically referred to the fact that a negative test does not imply no risk of disease. For example[e]:

> If the results of DNA testing are negative, the chance an individual has a
> CF [cystic fibrosis] gene is greatly diminished, but not eliminated. There
> are hundreds of mutations in the CF gene that can cause the disease. DNA
> tests identify only the most common mutations.[f]

For three key content elements, there were differences between materials from nonprofit and for-profit organizations: patient rights, the need for genetic counseling, and the purpose of the genetic test. Pamphlets from nonprofit organizations were likely to include information on patient rights, whereas none of the 21 pamphlets from for-profit organizations had such information (P<0.001) (see Table 2). Nonprofits were more likely to include the need for or availability of genetic counseling (P<0.001).

A typical example of a statement on patient rights in pamphlets from nonprofit organizations is, "All testing is voluntary and all information is confidential." A few pamphlets, however, had much lengthier statements including limitations on disclosure and confidentiality of family members:

---

[e]Because of the need for confidentiality, we identify pamphlets sources by disease only.
[f]Pamphlet on CF testing from nonprofit organization.

Your participation in this presymptomatic testing procedure is at your request, and you have the option to suspend or interrupt the testing procedure at any time. This diagnostic procedure will indicate only the likelihood of having inherited multiple endocrine neoplasia. DNA samples from your family will be sorted and used in the diagnosis of this disease only. Disclosure of testing results will be done only to the person being tested. Although the genetic data may be used in research studies, the identity of family members will be held in strict confidentiality, and will not be released except following written notification by a family member, in cases of medical emergency.[g]

A typical statement in pamphlets from nonprofit organizations on the need for genetic counseling is: "Genetic counseling is available to help families understand genetic testing and how the results might affect choices about health care."[h] Materials on tests for adult onset disorders such as Huntington disease, for which there is higher concern about psychosocial impacts of testing, however, often had more extensive statements, such as:

Testing involves education and counseling about the implications of the testing by someone with expertise in genetic testing such as a genetic counselor or medical geneticist. A neurological examination is also performed. Individuals with symptoms may discuss testing with a neurologist. A person with depression, changes in behavior, or psychiatric illness should also be seen by a psychologist or psychiatrist.[i]

Pamphlets from nonprofit organizations were, however, much less likely to specify the intended purpose of the test (i.e., as a screening, diagnostic, carrier and/or predictive test) ($P<0.0001$) (see Table 2). An example of such a specification in a pamphlet from a for-profit organization is:

What is the CF carrier test? There is now a test which can detect the most common disease-causing changes in the CF gene, and which therefore can find most of the people who are CF carriers.

SUMMARY AND CONCLUSIONS

- Overall, pamphlets tended to contain information that would aid in determining a patient's eligibility for a genetic test, but did not contain sufficient information about the tests themselves.
- Several critical elements need to be added to most pamphlets to enhance informed choices by patients and providers. Price lists with shipping information and general pamphlets on genetic diseases do not provide adequate information about the tests.

---

[g]Pamphlet from a nonprofit organization on inherited multiple endocrine neoplasia.
[h]Pamphlet concerning cystic fibrosis testing.
[i]Pamphlet on Huntington disease.

• Information about test performance should specify whether it refers to sensitivity or specificity (relative to a specified gold standard) or predictive value (in a specified population). Deficiencies in information on test interpretation are particularly serious given the high proportion of physicians who misinterpret test results.[31]

• Nonprofit organizations developing informational materials on genetic tests might consider enveloping pamphlets that are specifically aimed at patients, if they do not do so already. Their materials should add clear information about the intended purpose and uses of the relevant tests.

• Materials from for-profit organizations should add information on patients' rights, such as the voluntary and confidential nature of testing, the need for informed consent, and the need for and availability of genetic counseling. This information needs to be included in materials designed for providers as well as patients.

ACKNOWLEDGMENTS

We thank Stephen Hilgartner for help in developing the telephone survey questions and the criteria for content analysis. This study was supported in part by a grant from the Robert Wood Johnson Foundation (to N. A. H.)

ABOUT THE AUTHOR

Dr. Cho is an Assistant Professor of Bioethics at the University of Pennsylvania Center for Bioethics and the Department of Molecular and Cellular Engineering. She is a former Pew Health Policy fellow, and VA Health Services Research fellow. Any opinions expressed in this paper are those of the authors, and do not necessarily reflect those of the University of Pennsylvania.

REFERENCES

1. F. Giardiello, J. Brensinger, G. Petersen, M. Luce, L. Hylind, J. Bacon, S. Booker, R. Parker, S. Hamilton. The use and interpretation of commercial APC gene testing for familial adenomatous polyposis. *N Engl J Med* 336:823-7 (1997).

2. J. Harvey, R. Plumridge. Comparative attitudes to verbal and written medication information among hospital outpatients. *DICP* 25:925-928 (1991).

3. E. Clayton, V. Hanning, J. Pfotenhauer, R. Parker, P. Campbell, J. Phillips. Teaching about cystic fibrosis carrier screening by using written and video information. *Am J Hum Genet* 57:171-181 (1995).

4. V. Culbertson, T. Arthur, P. Rhodes, R. Rhodes. Consumer preferences for verbal and written medication information. *DICP* 22:390-396 (1988).

5. L.Laine, R. Shulman, K. Bartholomew, P. Gardner, T. Reed, S. Cole. An educational booklet diminishes anxiety in parents who*se* children receive total parental nutrition. Am J Dis Child 143:374-377 (1989).

6. Task Force on Genetic Testing. Interim Principles. (Baltimore, MD: 1996). Available at http://www.med.jhu.edu/tfgte/si.

7. P. Billings, M. Kohn, M. de Cuevas, J. Beckwith, J. Alper, M. Natowicz. Discrimination as a consequence of genetic testing. *Am J Hum Genet* 50:476-482 (1992).

8. T. Duster. Backdoor to Eugenics (New York: Routledge: 1990).

9. M. Natowicz, J. Alper, J. Alper. Genetic discrimination and the law. *Am J Hum Genet* 50:465-475 (1992).

10. D. Nelkin, L. Tancredi. Dangerous diagnostics: the social power of biological information. (New York: Basic Books, Inc. Publ.: 1989).

11. P. Reilly. Eugenic sterilization in the United States. In: A. Milunsky, G. Annas, eds. *Genetics and the Law III* pp. 227-241 (New York: Plenum: 1985).

12. D. Axworthy, D. Brock, M. Bobrow, T. Marteau. Psychological impact of population-based carrier testing for cystic fibrosis: 3-year follow-up. UK Cystic Fibrosis Follow-Up Study Group *Lancet* 347:1443-1446 (1996).

13. M. Bloch, S. Adam, S. Wiggins, M. Huggins, M. R. Hayden. Predictive testing for Huntington disease in Canada: The experience of those receiving an increased risk. *Am J Med Genet* 42:499-507 (1992).

14. A-M. Codori, J. Brandt. Psychological Costs and Benefits of Predictive Testing for Huntington's Disease. *Am J Med Genet (Neuropsychiatric Genetics)* 54:174-184 (1994).

15. A-M. Codori, R. Hanson, J. Brandt. Self-selection in predictive testing for Huntington's Disease. *Am J Med Genet* 54:167-173 (1994).

16. M. Huggins, M. Bloch, S. Wiggins, *et al.* Predictive Testing for Huntington Disease in Canada: Adverse Effects and Unexpected Results in Those Receiving a Decreased Risk. *Am J Med Genet* 42:508-515 (1992).

17. T. Thelin, E. McNeil, T. Aspegren-Jannson, T. Sveger. Psychological consequences of neonatal screening for alpha 1-antitrypsin deficiency (ATD). *Acta Paed Scand* 74:841-847 (1985).

18. American Society of Clinical Oncology Statement of the American Society of Clinical Oncology: genetic testing for cancer susceptibility. *J Clin Oncology* 14:1730-1736 (1996).

19. L. Andrews, J. Fullarton, N. Holtzman, A. Motulsky, eds. *Assessing genetic risks: implications for health and social policy* (Washington, DC: National Academy Press: 1993).

20. Committee on Inborn Errors of Metabolism. Genetic screening: programs, principles, and research (Washington, DC: National Academy of Sciences: 1975).

21. President's Commission for the Study of Ethical Problems in Medicine and Biomedical and Behavioral Research Screening and Counseling for Genetic Conditions: the ethical, social and legal implications of genetic screening, counseling, and education programs (Washington, DC: 1983).

22. M. K. Cho, M. Arruda, and N. A. Holtzman. Educational material about genetic tests: Does it provide key information for patients and providers? *Am J Med Genet* 73:314-320 (1997).

23. N. A. Holtzman and S. Hilgartner. State of the Art of Genetic Testing in the United States: Survey of Biotechnology Companies and Nonprofit Clinical Laboratories and Interviews of Selected Organizations. Task Force On Genetic Testing. *Appendix 3,. Promoting Safe and Effective Genetic Testing in the United States: Final Report.*

24. Task Force on Genetic Testing (1996).

25. American Society of Clinical Oncology (1996).

26. L. Andrews, J. Fullarton, N. Holtzman, A. Motulsky (1993).

27. Committee on Inborn Errors of Metabolism (1975).

28. President's Commission for the Study of Ethical Problems in Medicine and Biomedical and Behavioral Research (1983).

29. M. K. Cho, M. Arruda, and N. A. Holtzman. Quality of informational material disseminated about genetic diagnostic tests. *Am J Hum Genet* 59(4 supplement):A333 (1997).

30. M. K. Cho, *et al.* Educational material about genetic tests (1997).

31. F. Giardiello, *et al.* (1997).

TABLE 1

CRITERIA FOR CONTENT ANALYSIS

Criteria	Description of Criteria
Intended purpose of test	A statement about whether the test was intended for use as a screening, diagnostic, carrier, and/or predictive test
Test performance	A statement describing the sensitivity, specificity, predictive value, false positive or false negative rate of the test
Risks, limitations, and benefits	A statement about medical or social benefits or risks (risks including insurance or employment discrimination, or psychosocial risks)
Rights of patients	A statement that testing was voluntary, that testing or test results were confidential, that the patient could specify to whom results could be disclosed, or about the need for informed consent
Candidates for testing	A description of medical and/or family history criteria that indicate that an individual is appropriate for testing
Description of condition detected by test	A description of symptoms, characteristics, incidence, and/or inheritance patterns of the condition(s) detected by the test
Genetic counseling	A statement that genetic counseling is available or necessary to accompany testing
Interpretation of test results	A statement explaining risk for disease or reproductive risk for those with positive and negative test results
Treatment options	A description of treatment, prevention, or other medical management options for the condition being tested
Cost	Cost to patient

		Criteria included?	
TABLE 2			
CONTENT ELEMENTS ASSOCIATED WITH PROFIT STATUS OF ORGANIZATION			
Criteria	**Profit Status**	**No**	**Yes**
Intended purpose of test (P<0.0001)	nonprofit	80% (75/94)	20% (19/94)
	for-profit	33% (7/21)	67% (14/21)
Rights of patients (P<0.001)	nonprofit	65% (61/94)	35% (33/94)
	for-profit	100% (21/21)	0% (0/21)
Genetic counseling (P<0.001)	nonprofit	21% (20/94)	79% (74/94)
	for-profit	57% (12/21)	43% (9/21)

APPENDIX 5. THE HISTORY OF NEWBORN PHENYLKETONURIA SCREENING IN THE U.S.[a]

Diane B. Paul[b]

INTRODUCTION

Phenylketonuria (PKU) is a rare genetic disorder, with an incidence in the U.S., Britain, and most of Western Europe of between 1 in 11,000 and 1 in 15,000 births.[1] Virtually all newborns are tested for it in every American state, Canada, Australia, New Zealand, Japan, the nations of Western and most of Eastern Europe, and many other countries throughout the world. Normally, such a rare condition would not attract such attention, but PKU is a treatable genetic disease.

In the past, it generally resulted in severe mental retardation and behavioral and other abnormalities. About 90 percent of those affected had IQs of less than 50.[2,3,4] The symptoms of the disease result from a deficiency in a liver enzyme that catalyzes the conversion of phenylalanine (an essential amino acid that cannot be synthesized by humans) to tyrosine. In the absence of therapy, phenylalanine accumulates to toxic levels in the blood. Fortunately, mental retardation can be prevented and other symptoms mitigated if newborns are placed on a special diet from which most of the phenylalanine has been removed.

Thus, PKU screening provides an attractive example to proponents of genetic medicine and has come to be considered the "epitome of the application of human biochemical genetics," and a model for genetic medicine and public health.[5] Its appeal is partly explained by the dearth of other examples of effective interventions for genetic disorders. In general, advances in genetic knowledge have not been matched by corresponding progress in treatment (resulting in a "therapeutic gap").

At the same time, it demonstrates that "genetic" should not be equated with "unchangeable." PKU is an inborn error of metabolism, and it is our knowledge of its biochemistry that enables us to limit the supply of the damaging substrate and avoid or mitigate the symptoms of the disease. Thus, PKU also is frequently applauded by critics of genetic determinism, even when they are otherwise skeptical of the value of screening programs.[6,7]

Since PKU has acquired symbolic meaning to groups with disparate and even conflicting perspectives on policy issues in genetics, it is perhaps not surprising that accounts of screening and treatment have often been idealized. But the reality is quite complex.

Broad-based PKU screening began in 1963, when, following the invention of a vastly improved test to detect PKU in infants, Massachusetts became the first state to mandate screening—that is, to make screening of all newborns compulsory by law. The National Association for Retarded Children (NARC), an organization representing parents of retarded children and professionals in the field, advocated the screening and found that its application was very uneven. For example, in 1964, in Massachusetts maternity hospitals, virtually all infants were screened, but in thirty-two other states, fewer than half of the hospitals had instituted screening programs. The NARC proposed a model law, and, with officials of the Children's Bureau of the Department of Health, Education, and Welfare and of state departments of public health,[8] promoted mandatory screening.

[a]The Task Force commissioned this paper and reviewed an early draft of it. The views expressed in this paper are those of the author and do not necessarily reflect the views of the Task Force.
[b]University of Massachusetts at Boston

Health, Education, and Welfare and of state departments of public health,[8] promoted mandatory screening.

By 1975, forty-three states had enacted such laws and 90 percent of all newborns were being tested.[9] Today, every American state screens newborns for PKU and congenital hypothyroidism. Nearly all screen for additional metabolic disorders as well.[10] In only two states (Maryland and Wyoming) is explicit parental consent required for every screening program.[11]

Mandated screening was opposed by the American Medical Association and many state medical societies. More surprisingly, compulsory screening was also opposed rather quietly by many researchers in the field of human metabolism. For a variety of reasons, these researchers believed it premature to mandate that every infant be tested for PKU and their reservations intensified during the first few years of the screening programs.[12,13,14,15,16,17]

By almost any standard, though, PKU screening counts as a success. At relatively low cost, it has prevented mental retardation in thousands of infants worldwide. It is a significant achievement that these individuals and their families have been spared the devastating effects of the disease. But treatment has not been easy to manage, has not been completely efficacious, and has greatly exacerbated the problem of "maternal PKU."

It is of special interest that many of the problems accompanying screening and treatment were in fact anticipated by human metabolic researchers.

PKU SCREENING: THE EARLY YEARS

As early as the 1930s, biochemists George Jervis and Richard Block in the U.S. and Lionel Penrose in Britain proposed treating affected infants with a low-phenylalanine diet.[18,19,20] But for a number of reasons (including assumptions about the cost of producing the synthetic food), these early proposals were not pursued.

The idea that a phenylalanine-restricted diet could prevent or diminish symptoms associated with PKU was revived in 1951 by English biochemists Louis Woolf and David Vulliamy.[21] Woolf and colleagues tested the theory on three small children, all of whom showed some improvement.[22] Other researchers in Britain and the U.S. reported improvement in small numbers of older infants and children treated with a low-phenylalanine diet.[23,24,25,26,27] Although the first retrospective statistical study assessing the benefits of dietary therapy would not appear until 1960,[28] these reports generated great excitement for they held out hope that mental retardation, then considered therapeutically hopeless, might in fact be treatable.[29]

Notwithstanding some early claims that dietary therapy markedly increased the IQs of severely retarded children so that they might even be able to attend school, it was becoming increasingly clear that once retardation occurred, it could not be reversed.[30,31] Reviewing the experience between 1950 and 1959 with dietary therapy, Horst Bickel and Werner Grueter noted that the chances of cognitive improvement were greatest in the youngest patients and concluded: "Every effort should be made to start the diet in early infancy, if possible, within the first few months of life."[32] Identification of the infants with PKU would require population-wide screening (unless testing were restricted to the newborn siblings of previously affected children, a pool containing only a small proportion of all cases).[33] These considerations, and the availability of Lofenalac, a commercially-available formula approved by the FDA in 1958 (based on experience with just six patients) prompted some hospitals, clinics, and private physicians to begin testing newborns for the disease.

However, the ferric chloride urine test, then the only method available, was unreliable until the age of six to eight weeks, after the infant had been discharged from the hospital and possibly after he or she had already suffered some irreversible brain damage. It was thus unsuitable for mass screening.

In 1960, the microbiologist Robert Guthrie (who had a mentally retarded son and niece, the latter diagnosed with PKU) developed an inexpensive, sensitive, and simple bacterial inhibition assay that could be administered a few days after birth. At the urging of the President and the Executive Director of the NARC, he published his report on the test quickly, as a letter to the editor, so that it could be publicized in connection with the NARC's 1961 poster featuring two little sisters with PKU.[34] This mode of announcement, and the fact that a peer-reviewed report on the test was not published until 1963 [35] led to some tensions with the community of human metabolic researchers. The situation was exacerbated when Guthrie—an outsider to the community—took his case directly to parents, legislators, and the press.

In late 1961, the Children's Bureau began a field trial involving over 400,000 infants in 29 states to assess the assay's suitability for a national screening program. By the time the trial ended in 1963, the Bureau had adopted the slogan, "Test Every Newborn For PKU."

Development of the Guthrie test converged with new thinking about the intractable problem of mental retardation. During the 1950s, public and private agencies had begun to reconsider their traditional emphasis on educational, social, and rehabilitative services for the retarded. A turn toward scientific prevention appeared increasingly attractive to government agencies, legislators, and the NARC.[36] The hope was that "the same scientific methods which have accomplished so much in the conquest of other diseases can now be harnessed to the study of mental defects."[37]

Even before development of the Guthrie test, this shift in emphasis was accompanied by strong claims for the significance of screening programs. In spite of its rarity, the prevention of PKU was portrayed as a means to substantially reduce the frequency of retardation. For example, the *New York Times* (April 7, 1957) explained the emphasis on early detection of retardation in a new government program for the preschool mentally retarded on the grounds that "much" mental retardation results from the treatable hereditary diseases, PKU and (the even rarer) galactosemia.

In 1961, President John F. Kennedy (whose sister Rosemary was mentally retarded) announced a major federal initiative. He promised to double the amount spent by the National Institutes of Health on retardation research, and appointed a Presidential Advisory Commission on Mental Retardation, charging it with appraising the adequacy of existing programs in the field. The Commission included major proponents of the scientific approach to the prevention of retardation and their perspective was reflected in its 1962 recommendations. Thus, newborn screening programs were characterized as an "important" step in preventing mental retardation and their expansion was recommended, even though the only screening experience at this time involved the unsatisfactory—and for that reason, generally discarded—ferric chloride urine test.[38]

The Commission also hired the Advertising Council to publicize the magnitude of the problem of retardation (an effort financed jointly by the Department of Health, Education, and Welfare and the Joseph P. Kennedy Foundation). The Advertising Council mounted a dramatic campaign advocating that the new PKU test "should be a must for all babies everywhere."

Lamenting that only Massachusetts, New York, Louisiana, and Rhode Island mandated testing, the ads compared the 50¢ [unit] cost of the test with the $100,000 required for lifetime care of institutionalized victims of the disease, and asserted—without any supporting evidence—that with a special diet, "a PKU baby then grows and develops as normally as any other child." They also urged citizens in states without legislation to demand that their states make testing of all infants compulsory.[39]

A member of the Children's Bureau staff protested futilely that "the proposals seemed in advance of general medical readiness" and went well beyond the recommendations of the Academy of Pediatrics.[40]

Even before the field trial had ended, the Guthrie test was being hailed as a major discovery, with the potential to reduce both the suffering and the financial burden associated with the disease. In numerous newspaper and magazine articles, it was described as an achievement with a potentially vast impact on mental retardation—though in the U.S., universal newborn PKU screening identifies fewer than 400 cases each year.

Screening was even promoted as a means to reduce overcrowding in institutions for the mentally retarded. After noting that there were approximately 5 ½ million mentally retarded individuals in the United States, Senator Joseph Montoya asserted that: "Many of these are a result of phenylketonuria and their mental retardation could have been prevented if detected in infancy. Most of the State training schools for the mentally retarded are overcrowded and have long waiting lists for admission".[41] However, it had long been known that PKU was the cause of retardation in less than one percent of institutionalized patients [42] and a 1962 Children's Bureau census had identified only 399 children with PKU admitted to programs for the mentally retarded during the preceding five years. The relatively few beds once occupied by patients with PKU would certainly be filled quickly with other severely impaired individuals.

Even commentators who acknowledged the rarity of the disease often considered screening a breakthrough, for they viewed it as a model for the prevention of other diseases. "The ailment is rare, but its importance is not to be measured in terms of numbers alone," wrote Harold Schmeck Jr. in the *New York Times* of May 21, 1961, explaining that its primary value was as a model for elucidating the causes of other disorders, especially those causing mental deficiency. The significance of PKU was often implicitly equated with the significance of mental retardation. In a typical passage, a writer for the *Family Weekly* noted that PKU "strikes only one child in 20,000. But circumventing this disease has opened a way toward eradicating the blight of mental retardation which, in the United States alone, afflicts 5,500,000 persons."[43] Guthrie himself argued that "the conquest of PKU is important not only for itself, but because it serves as an open door to a whole new era of preventive medicine based upon new understanding of medical genetics" (quoted in *Parents' Magazine,* Nov. 1995, p. 108). Contemporary assumptions concerning the potential impact of the Guthrie test were reflected in the American Medical Association's 1962 year-end report, which cited it (along with the unraveling of the genetic code) as a major medical breakthrough.

In the 1960s, it was assumed that early dietary treatment of some form would prevent complications in most other inherited metabolic disorders and some writers assumed it would prevent other forms of mental retardation and/or mental illness. Referring to galactosemia, cystic fibrosis of the pancreas, glycogen storage disease, and idiopathic hyperlipemia, one author wrote: "These diseases can now be readily diagnosed and controlled by changes in diet."[44] Another explained that the discovery of an organic cause for PKU "suggests that, in time, certain other mental ailments—including schizophrenia and manic-depressive psychosis—may be found to have similar roots.[45]

Bolstered by this confidence in the efficacy of dietary treatment for many disorders, newborn screening initially appeared a much more powerful tool in combating retardation than, unfortunately, it turned out in practice to be. Readers of *Good Housekeeping* (Feb. 1966, p. 177) were assured that if dietary therapy were begun early enough, "a child will develop to his full mental potential." But in 1966, no one could possibly know if this claim were true. Relatively few early-treated infants had reached an age when their adult cognitive functioning could be predicted.[46] In 1965, a committee of the American Academy of Pediatrics noted that since an adequate diet had only become available in 1958 and early screening tests into general use after 1960, only a few individuals had been diagnosed with PKU within the first month of life, and "even they have been treated for less than six years, and this period of time is inadequate for assessing child development and projecting eventual intellectual ability on optimum treatment."[47] In addition, the developmental tests administered to infants and young children emphasized sensory and motor skills, not verbal and conceptual ones.[48] These tests could only be very imperfect instruments for predicting infants' ultimate intellectual achievement.

SKEPTICAL VOICES

As the above discussion suggests, there were also skeptical voices—some loud and some muted. One of the most vocal and extreme of the scientific critics was biochemist Samuel Bessman. Some of his concerns were shared by more circumspect colleagues, but he also argued, contra the scientific consensus, that the intelligence of "many" individuals with PKU would be normal without any treatment; that the apparent benefits of dietary therapy could well be attributed to placebo effects, and that the abnormalities associated with the disease were more likely to result from a deficiency of tyrosine than an excess of phenylalanine.[49,50,51]

Howard University political scientist Joseph Cooper was another emphatic critic. He publicized Bessman's views in articles, lectures, and testimony at legislative hearings, but he spoke for himself, rather than Bessman, when he charged that the emphasis on scientific prevention would deflect attention from much more pressing problems of the mentally retarded.[52,53] Noting that the vast majority of mentally retarded individuals did not suffer from PKU, or indeed any genetic defect, Cooper argued that their greatest need was for social support, not science. "What are we doing," he asked, "about the home-situated retardees who awaken one day to find that their parents or relatives are gone or no longer able to care for them? What do we do about these people? They must certainly outnumber those with PKU."[54] (Paul Edelson has argued that screening did indeed have the effect of moving social policy away from the provision of educational and social services to scientific prevention—a way of framing the issue that had little, if any, relevance to the vast majority of mentally retarded Americans.[55])

Most PKU researchers, including Bessman, focused on a narrower set of issues. One issue concerned the sensitivity and specificity of the Guthrie test. It was originally assumed that the results of Guthrie blood testing would be compared with later, more definitive tests. Guthrie himself suggested that tests be run both on the blood collected in the hospital and on urine-impregnated filter papers, which the mother would mail back to the laboratory when the infant was 2 to 3 weeks old. He assumed that this method would avoid frequent false positives,[56,57] but the follow-up urine test soon proved unsatisfactory.[58,59]

The consultants to the California state health department expressed reservations shared by many researchers when they complained that data submitted on the Guthrie test were inadequate for determining either its specificity or sensitivity and expressed concern that some infants with confirmed high phenylalanine levels at 2 to 3 weeks might not require dietary treatment. Eight of nine consultants agreed that, although the test promised to be much more satisfactory than the ferric chloride test, "it requires further evaluation and our knowledge of PKU needs to be more complete before mass trials on the basis proposed by Dr. Guthrie would be justified." The consultants concluded "that more effective studies and approaches to PKU and screening procedures could be conducted by focusing on high risk populations and by more intensive studies in several areas as contrasted to deploying practically all available resources in a mass Guthrie Inhibition Assay screening procedure."[60]

The first systematic effort to assess the accuracy of the test did not appear until 1974. It reported that about 10 percent of infants with PKU were being missed by screening (either because they were not tested or because the test did not detect PKU), while only 5.1 percent of presumptively positive screening tests were confirmed as "classical PKU" (defined as a blood phenylalanine level of 20 mg/100 ml or more) on retesting.[61]

Guthrie had considered false positives a "small cost" in comparison with the benefit derived from early detection. That conclusion reflected a common assumption (now as then) that the costs in time, money, stress, and possibility of unneeded treatment are much less significant than the harm due to missed cases of the disease. On this assumption, screening tests should be oversensitive, so that all true cases are identified. "Although false positive tests [for inborn errors of metabolism] are acceptable within defined limits," wrote Harold Nitowsky, "there should be no false negative tests."[62]

Initial screening positives were confirmed with column and paper amino acid chromatography, the fluorimetric assay for phenylalanine, or a second Guthrie blood test (the last allowing the test to be its own criterion for accuracy) although Guthrie himself stressed that a positive Guthrie test "should be confirmed by repeated tests upon new blood specimens, and also by at least one independent method of determining blood phenylalanine."[63]

Testing uncovered many more apparent cases of PKU than would have been predicted on the basis of studies of the institutionalized mentally retarded. Studies of populations of retarded patients seemed to indicate that the frequency of PKU was between 1 in 20,000 and 1 in 25,000 individuals of European ancestry. But the results of Guthrie testing in Massachusetts indicated that it was actually about 1 in 14,000. Mabry, Nelson, and Horner argued that some part of the discrepancy was explained by hyperphenylalaninemic infants who were not retarded.[64] But while it was evident to most researchers that elevated blood phenylalanine levels could result from conditions other than classical PKU, no one knew what proportion of these individuals were actually at risk of retardation.

The problem of variant forms led to enormous confusion in the interpretation of elevated blood phenylalanine levels in newborns and its subsequent treatment. Guthrie and many pediatricians continued to believe that anyone with a slight but persistently above-normal phenylalanine level was at risk for retardation. But Berman, *et al.* found that older siblings of infants with elevated blood phenylalanine under 20 mg/100 ml levels also had moderate elevations but normal mental development.[65] Most researchers argued that infants with moderate elevations were at no risk for retardation and should not be treated. In 1980, O'Flynn *et al.* found that 20 of 195 infants with markedly elevated phenylalanine levels on screening had variant forms that probably did not require treatment.[66] (But for recent challenges to the view that moderate elevations of phenylalanine are safe, see Guttler *et al.* 1993[67] and Diamond 1994.[68])

Uncertainty about who needed to be treated led to concern that some infants without PKU were being damaged by the diet. Some researchers believed that little harm would come from treating such infants. Woolf believed that twice as many patients were being treated for PKU as might be necessary but considered the financial cost, need to adhere to an unpalatable diet, and danger of dietary deficiencies "a small price to pay for preventing the mental deterioration otherwise inevitable in at least half of them".[69] Others thought that unnecessary treatment could itself produce mental retardation.[70] Several reports of deaths and diet-deficiency syndromes suffered by infants on PKU diets led researchers also to fear that some infants with the disease were being harmed by too-drastic treatment or suffering severe malnutrition as the result of diet refusal.[71] Problems in dietary management were compounded by uncertainty over the optimal level of phenylalanine and the exact phenylalanine content of foods and by the unpalatability of the special diet.

Moreover, there was no consensus as to how long treatment was needed. Some researchers assumed that only infants and young children needed to maintain the restricted diet.[72] They thought that when gross brain development was complete (around the age of five), it would be possible for children to eat normally. Others thought that therapy should be continued longer, even through adolescence.[73,74]

In articles and reports intended for nonspecialists, the more optimistic assumption was often presented as undoubted fact; the public was told that children could be taken off the diet by the age of five or six "for no further damage can occur once the brain is fully developed".[75,76]

Skeptical researchers also noted that intensive social and psychological support services would be required if dietary therapy were to be effective and predicted that these problems would be exacerbated if it turned out that the diet had to be maintained beyond early childhood. In short, they argued that too little was known about the nature of the disease, the reliability of the test, or the efficacy of treatment to justify compulsory screening.

Proponents, on the other hand, noted that, prior to the enactment of mandated screening laws, some states had low levels of participation and they argued that, in respect to the others, missing even one child was too great a cost. While generally conceding that there were many unknowns in the diagnosis and treatment of PKU, they maintained (in the words of Robert MacCready, Director of the Massachusetts Public Health Department and Chair of the Public Health Committee of the NARC) that "just as we must go into the water to learn to swim, we must continue to search out, treat, and study the phenylketonurics." They also stressed the importance of PKU screening as a "breakthrough prototype," asserting that it was "bound to progress toward control of the other inborn errors of metabolism associated with mental retardation."[77]

But even within the Children's Bureau, concerns mounted that screening might have been routinized prematurely. Bessman's claim that once legislation and fear of malpractice suits had combined to make treatment universal, it would be difficult and perhaps impossible to learn the answers to important scientific questions, resonated with some researchers. Members of the Bureau's Ad Hoc Committee on Medical Genetics reflected this concern when they suggested "that alternate cases of tyrosinemia be treated to learn whether there is value in therapy before medico-legal problems, which have arisen in PKU, prevent an objective and scientific evaluation of the treatment of this metabolic disease also."[78] (On discussions concerning mass screening for tyrosinemia and also Wilson's disease, see Swazey 1971).[79]

A very small randomized clinical trial (RCT), in which only seven infants did not receive the special diet, would have sufficed to establish its efficacy.[80] But it was impossible to mount such a trial given the claims of benefit. (Although RCTs are more popular today than they were in the 1960s, most bioethicists consider withholding a treatment considered efficacious by a majority of researchers to violate the principle of "equipoise."[81]) In 1967, the Children's Bureau funded, as an alternative, the United States Collaborative Study of children treated for phenylketonuria (PKUCS)—a project that involved nineteen centers across the U.S. in following (originally) 224 infants diagnosed with PKU as a result of newborn screening. The PKUCS represented a systematic effort to investigate the effectiveness of dietary treatment by treating all infants, but to varying degree. It demonstrated that the diet was adequate for normal physical growth, could result in near-normal levels of intelligence, should be maintained throughout childhood, and that the most important factor in predicting IQ was the age at which the low phenylalanine diet is begun.[82]

SCREENING IN PRACTICE: A BRIEF SUMMARY

Initial problems of high false negative and very high false positive rates and unreliable laboratory work were eventually solved. But all the initial assumptions about the ease and effectiveness of therapy turned out to be much too sanguine and new problems emerged. The literature on cognitive and neuropsychological outcomes is vast: what follows is a very brief summary.

While nutritional therapy prevents retardation, intellectual deficits and psychosocial problems are common. Even early and well treated individuals with phenylketonuria often have lower IQs than would normally be expected and may experience other deficits; these include learning disabilities, visual/motor difficulties, increased emotional lability, agoraphobia, and thought disorders.[83,84,85,86,87,88,89,90,91] As a consequence, individuals with PKU often require long-term medical, social, psychological, and rehabilitative services.

The most serious deficits result from failure to maintain strict dietary control. Studies eventually revealed that IQ scores declined after the diet was abandoned; as a consequence, dietary recommendations became progressively more conservative. According to Virginia Schuett, recent reports prove that "high blood phenylalanine levels are not safe for anyone; they never have been, they never will be."[92] While not everyone agrees with the need for "diet for life,"[93,94] most treatment centers in the U.S. now do recommend lifelong continuance—a goal that is not easy to achieve.

DIETARY MANAGEMENT

Many accounts of screening assume an inevitable bridge between diagnosis and treatment. However, strict adherence to the diet is extremely difficult to achieve, especially in adolescents. The PKU diet involves phenylalanine-free or reduced substitutes for most natural protein foods, including bread, cake, meat, fish, eggs, and dairy products[95] supplemented by a formula with extra tyrosine and

144

other amino acids, vitamins, and minerals. For a number of reasons, most individuals with PKU (and their families) find the diet extremely taxing and few fully comply with it.

The formula is unpalatable, both the formula and special phenylalanine-free foods are burdensome to prepare, and the diet as a whole is boring. Adhering to it requires considerable motivation and skill. Even generally high-functioning individuals with PKU often suffer from math deficits, which makes diet calculations difficult. The formula and special foods are also expensive—roughly $5,000 per year for the formula alone.

Unfortunately, there are few studies of who pays for the diet therapy and how. We do know that there is tremendous variation in the quality and extent of services provided (as expected in state-based programs). However, while forty-three states had passed screening laws by 1975, none mandated treatment. Even now, many states neither provide treatment nor require insurers to reimburse for it.[96] Some states require reimbursement for treatment for PKU but not for other metabolic disorders; some provide for treatment "where practicable" or if the budget allows.[97]

In the early years of the program, the states generally subsidized the formula for infants and children (and continue to do so) and children were generally taken off-diet at the age of five or six. Moreover, the formula was originally classified as a drug, and was reimbursable for those with health insurance. When it lost this status in 1972, many insurers came to treat it as a food and refused to reimburse. At the same time, adolescents and even adults were increasingly advised to remain on-diet. While some states have passed laws requiring insurance companies to pay for the diet, self-insurers, who provide at least half of employee health insurance, are exempt from state laws under the Employee Retirement Income Security Act.

A study of the situation in New York, based on the experience of patients at three metabolic disorders treatment centers, is discouraging. Although half of the patients were covered by private health insurance and a quarter by Medicaid, most were unable to obtain reimbursement from these sources. The author writes: "The centers reported that many families considered the cost of these special foods to be a major burden. Their staffs interceded for patients by appealing to private insurance carriers and to local Medicaid offices to attempt to reverse decisions which had denied reimbursement for special foods. They reported that their efforts were rarely effective."[98]

In general, insurers have little knowledge of PKU (or any rare genetic disorder). Thus it is often necessary to explain, protest, provide extra documentation—a process that is especially wearing on families that already have problems coping with the disease.[99] Providers and health departments, who often make Herculean efforts to help, know that "the fact that effective therapy exists . . . does not mean that it is actually accessible to the children who need it."[100]

Even without the financial problems of supplying the diet, there are difficulties with compliance. Food is integral to religious and ethnic identity—which explains why immigrants' food habits are the last to change. Eating the same foods is one way of showing that we belong to a group.[101] Not surprisingly, women with PKU find it particularly hard to cope with holiday celebrations, which are frequently linked to religious and ethnic identity and often focus on food.[102]

Most important, meals express friendship and are used to establish intimacy.[103] Individuals who must avoid common foods face profound barriers to eating with others. They find it awkward to explain their dietary restrictions, know from experience that even if they do, people sometimes forget and they will be served something they should not eat, and that their friends and relatives will often assume that it's fine if you only eat a little of the restricted food item. These difficult choices and embarrassing situations are particularly hard on adolescents, who are insecure and especially susceptible to advertising and peer pressure.[104] In the literature on insulin-dependent diabetes mellitus, there is a consensus "that adolescents as a group display the worst metabolic control."[105] Indeed, the folk wisdom seems to be that no adolescent fully adheres to the diabetic diet—which is considerably less burdensome than the diet for PKU.

Moreover, noncompliance with all medical advice is in general more likely when treatment recommendations are preventive rather than curative and when they involve lifestyle changes.[106] For all these (and other) reasons, eating behavior is very resistant to change. When it comes to young women with PKU, that is an especially serious problem.[107] For if they do not resume the diet prior to conception and maintain it throughout pregnancy, the effects on their offspring may be catastrophic.

THE PROBLEM OF MATERNAL PKU

Infants born to women with PKU do not themselves usually have the disease. However, high concentrations of phenylalanine are teratogenic—and the phenylalanine circulating in the maternal blood of women with PKU easily crosses the placental barrier. As a result, the offspring of women with classical PKU who do not maintain good dietary control are at great risk of mental retardation and microcephaly (over 90 percent) and lower risk (12-15 percent) for congenital birth defects and other anomalies.[108]

It is not easy for anyone to stay on the restrictive diet, much less to resume it. It is especially difficult during pregnancy when it is also necessary to consume about 25 percent more of the formula. Moreover, even well-functioning women with PKU often do not know how to cook.[109] As Charles Scriver writes: "It is possible to normalize the maternal metabolic phenotype during pregnancy with benefit to the fetus, [but] the effort required to achieve these goals can be awesome."[110]

Before the advent of newborn screening, women with PKU were severely retarded and often institutionalized so that they bore very few children. Most young women today discontinued the diet during childhood and have not been followed for many years. Since their fertility is now nearly normal, screening has had the paradoxical effect of converting a rare occurrence into a major problem.[111] Indeed, all the social benefits of screening may be neutralized by the birth of retarded children to women who have ended the diet.[112]

The Maternal PKU Collaborative Study (MPKUCS), which began in 1984, identified 402 pregnancies; researchers found that few of the young women were on diet (101 had IQs lower than 80). There were so few preconceptually treated and well-controlled pregnancies when the study began that researchers were unable to determine whether the current diet provides for adequate fetal growth and development.[113]

There are also some grounds for optimism. The socio-economic status and intellectual ability of the women enrolled in the study have improved over time. There has been a significant drop in the number of teenage pregnancies. And more women are initiating the diet preconceptually.[114]

Today, it is commonly said that the problem of maternal PKU came to attention as a result of the screening's success.

In fact, there were efforts in the early 1960s to focus attention on the potential problem. A report of three mentally retarded (nonphenylketonuric) offspring born to a woman with PKU appeared even before mass screening began[115] and in 1963, higher profile warnings appeared in *The New England Journal of Medicine*[116] and the *Journal of Pediatrics*.[117] Other discussions followed.[118,119,120,121]

But neither these discussions nor an editorial in the *New England Journal of Medicine*[122] had much impact. Legislators were surely unaware of the issues; indeed, in some states, screening laws passed by acclamation or voice vote and without either hearings or floor debates.[123] Robert Guthrie tried to prompt the Children's Bureau to action but even he was unsuccessful. Ironically, one reason seems to have been staffers' determination, in light of earlier experience, not to act prematurely.[124]

SCREENING FOR OTHER METABOLIC DISORDERS

Because PKU is such a rare disease (whose incidence also varies with ethnicity), some early screening programs identified few, if any, cases. Thus, in the first three years of the Washington, DC, program, no infants with PKU were identified and officials reasoned that they had better things to do with their money. Some other jurisdictions threatened to follow Washington's example and end their programs. The paucity of cases combined with problems that emerged in the first years of screening prompted a reappraisal of the value of screening programs.

One response was to load more tests on the original. By the end of the 1960s, a variety of other rare metabolic disorders were being detected with the same filter paper blood specimen employed for PKU screening. Most of these disorders could not be treated as effectively as PKU and at least one (histidinemia) was benign.

In the 1970s, a number of efforts were made to appraise the early history of PKU screening. All drew a similar lesson: there should be no rush to new screening programs. Thus, a committee of the National Research Council urged legislatures to avoid "*ad hoc* responses to pleas for state involvement in the increasing number of conditions for which screening will become available".[125] Harold Nitowsky spoke for many analysts when he wrote:

> I believe that we shall be forced to the conclusion that our knowledge of the natural history and variability of PKU is incomplete, that the effectiveness of treatment of the disease has not been accurately measured, that we have inadequate information about the optimal age for institution of dietary therapy, or the levels of serum phenylalanine (PA) at which treatment should be undertaken, or the age at which treatment may be stopped. Despite these unanswered questions, and the obvious lack of adequate validation of prescriptive screening, I do not believe we should turn backwards. . . . However, the lessons we have learned from our experiences with this disorder should serve as a warning against any impulsive or premature extension of prescriptive screening to a variety of other inborn errors of metabolism which are associated with serious illness or mental retardation, and for which screening tests are available as well as the possibility of dietary control.[126]

In spite of such warnings and more formal statements of principle, new tests were added without even the degree of pilot testing to which the Guthrie test was subjected. Newborn screening is administered by the states, so the testing programs vary tremendously. Today, all states test for PKU and for congenital hypothyroidism, while 42 test for sickle-cell anemia and 38 for galactosemia. Only five test for tyrosinemia, three for cystic fibrosis, and two for toxoplasmosis. In general, the new tests have been added casually, with little systematic assessment of their value and risks, and also with little concern for obtaining informed consent.[127]

A NOTE ON COST-BENEFIT ARGUMENTS

PKU screening had originally been made mandatory partly out of concern that voluntary programs might cease to be cost-effective. Advocates stressed the financial benefits, and used cost-benefit arguments to bolster them. In the 1960s, such analyses often compared the expense of laboratory testing and evaluation and of treatment with the assumed expenses to the state of providing institutionalized care (typically for 20 or 25 years) for a portion of the affected infants and medical and hospital costs for those not institutionalized. The "expense of laboratory testing" was sometimes equated with the unit cost of the test rather than the cost of the program to identify one affected individual—perhaps because the latter would include the cost of retesting the large number of false positives that is involved in all screening for very rare conditions.[128]

Well into the 1970s, simplistic claims abounded. The following passage from a 1977 NIH publication is typical:

- PKU...occurs approximately once in every 14,000 births.
- Screening newborns for the disease costs $1.25 per test; thus, approximately $17,000 is spent to detect each case.
- An additional $8,000 to $16,000 must then be spent for dietary treatment over a 5 to 10 year period, to prevent the retarding effects of the disease. This brings the total cost of prevention to about $33,000 per child.
- Untreated, severe mental retardation care for, say, 50 years in an institution at a cost of $20 a day, would run to $365,000, more than 10 times the cost of prevention.
- Add to this saving the input from the treated individual through earnings, taxes, and family and societal contributions.
- Such figures must be convincing, for 48 states now require screening of newborns for PKU and other genetic diseases.

While no reputable econometric study would make such claims, the NIH report reflects the reasoning that informed many cost-benefit arguments, especially those aimed at the public and at federal and state legislators.

Such analyses ignore the distribution of costs among the various payers, and aggregate all of them, whether costs are assumed by individual families, insurers, or the state, although the cost burdens may vary widely. They do not take into account indirect and intangible harms, such as the anxiety produced by false positive tests, the stresses on families of managing the restrictive diet, and the costs associated with maternal PKU. Further, it is misleading to equate the averted costs of institutionalization for PKU with the average annual cost per institutionalized patient. Preventing the mental retardation associated with PKU would produce no more than a one percent drop in the inpatient population. The costs of the institutions are mostly fixed, so such a small patient reduction is unlikely to lead to an equivalent cost reduction.[129,130]

Cost-benefit considerations have, in the past, contributed to the trend to add new tests. An additional test adds only a marginal cost, since the same system can be used for collecting and transporting specimens and recording and reporting results. Thus, as Charles Scriver noted, "screening tests with relatively low yield can be included economically in such programs."[131]

This is not to imply that the costs of screening outweigh the benefits—on the contrary. A number of studies have shown that the cost to improve the outcome of PKU by screening and early treatment is comparable to other widely-used and accepted programs to prevent diseases or their manifestations.[132] Moreover, there are other non-institutional costs associated with having a child with mental retardation, including anxiety, stress, and continued expenses for medical and social care, and many medical interventions bring new problems in their trains; PKU is hardly unique in that respect. But these remarks do suggest that some considerations have been systematically ignored, thus distorting the ratio of benefits to costs.[133]

CONCLUSION

The history of PKU shows that it is easy to exaggerate the ease and efficacy of treatment and to understate the costs. It was said that dietary therapy would be inexpensive, brief, and easy to manage. Unfortunately, it is none of these. PKU has turned out to be a difficult chronic disease. The American medical system is oriented toward curing acute illnesses, not helping people with chronic ones to live well. Thus, it is relatively easier to obtain access to expensive diagnostic tests than help with activities of daily living. Assistance with such ordinary requirements is what many individuals with PKU need to function in their communities and to adhere to the diet. In maternal PKU, the amount of social support better predicts compliance with the diet than does IQ or knowledge.[134] Thus, effective treatment requires a focus on matters that lie outside the conventional bounds of medicine. PKU programs have come to pay much attention to the process of managing infants, children, and young adults, including pregnant women. That is presumably one reason that teenage pregnancies are down and IQs up. And it is a very important development. But as Friedman et al.[135] have recently warned, "unless adequate services and insurance to cover care of these pregnancies is firmly established, the ominous prediction of Kirkman" [who warned that all the gains of screening could be erased by the birth of infants to women with untreated PKU][136] may still come to pass.

Further, this history shows that once newborn screening programs became established, they may be rapidly routinized and, once routinized, easily expanded for other purposes. Human metabolic researchers had reservations, but with few exceptions, kept them to themselves. Even when they voiced doubts, it did not slow the approval of the screening programs. Thus, legislators heard only a chorus of good news. The newspapers and magazines they read made screening appear a major breakthrough in the battle against mental retardation, one that would be followed by prevention of other disorders. No wonder that, in most states, screening laws were passed without dissent—and that it was (and is) extremely easy to add new tests, even for diseases less treatable than PKU and after even less rigorous processes of validation.

149

Thus, a "technological imperative"[137] has combined with unrealistic assumptions about benefits to drive the expansion of screening programs. The lesson that such wholesale expansion is unwarranted has been repeatedly drawn since the early 1960s. Surely it is time to heed it.

ACKNOWLEDGMENTS

This report was based in part on research supported by the National Science Foundation under Grant No. SBR-9511909. An early draft was much improved by a critique by members of the Task Force on Genetic Testing; I am especially grateful for the extensive and constructive comments by its Chair, Neil A. Holtzman. All my work on newborn screening has benefitted from association with physician/historian Paul Edelson, and with the enormously dedicated members of the PKU CORPS at Children's Hospital, Boston. However, members of the CORPS are not responsible for the views expressed in this report, some of which they may well not share.

ABOUT THE AUTHOR

Diane B. Paul is Professor of Political Science and Co-director of the Program in Science, Technology, and Values at the University of Massachusetts at Boston and Research Associate in the Museum of Comparative Zoology at Harvard University. She has been an Exxon Fellow at MIT, a fellow of the Wissenschaftskolleg zu Berlin, a Resident Fellow of the Humanities Research Institute of the University of California, and the recipient of grants from the National Endowment for the Humanities and the National Science Foundation. Any opinions, findings, and conclusions or recommendations expressed in this paper are those of the author and do not necessarily reflect the views of the National Science Foundation.

REFERENCES

1. Editorial *Lancet* 337:1256-1257 (May 25,1991).

2. K. N. F. Shaw. Biochemical aspects of phenylketonuria. In: *The Clinical Team Looks at Phenylketonuria*. Children's Bureau, U.S. Dept. of Health, Education, and Welfare. (Washington, D.C.: U. S. Government Printing Office: 1964).

3. K. L. Acuff and R. R. Faden. A history of prenatal and newborn screening programs: lessons for the future. In: R. R. Faden, G. Geller, and M. Powers. *AIDS, Women, and the Next Generation.* p. 64 (New York: Oxford University Press:1991).

4. Committee on Genetics, American Academy of Pediatrics Newborn Screening Fact Sheets. *Pediatr* 98:490 (1996).

5. C. R. Scriver. Phenylketonura—genotypes and phenotypes. New Engl J Med 324:1280-1281 (May 2, 1991).

6. D. Nelkin and L. Tancredi. *Dangerous Diagnostics: The Social Power of Biological Information.* p. 160 (New York: Basic Books: 1989).

7. R. Hubbard and E. Wald. *Exploding the Gene Myth.* pp. 198-99 (Boston: Beacon Press: 1993).

8. National Research Council, Committee for the Study of Inborn Errors of Metabolism *Genetic Screening: Programs, Principles, and Research.* pp. 44-87 (Washington, D.C.: National Academy of Science: 1975).

9. National Research Council, Committee for the Study of Inborn Errors of Metabolism (1975).

10. Committee on Genetics, American Academy of Pediatrics. pp. 474, 484, 491 (1996).

11. E. H. Hiller, G. Landenburger, and M. K. Natowicz. Public participation in medical policy making and the status of consumer autonomy: The example of newborn screening programs in the United States. *Am J Pub Hlth* 87:1280-1288 (1997).

12. J. A. Anderson and K. F. Swaiman. *Phenylketonuria and Allied Metabolic Disorders.* Summary. Proceedings of a conference held at Washington, D.C. April 6-8, 1966. p. 238 (Washington, D.C.: U.S. Government Printing Office: 1967).

13. H. K. Berry, and S. Wright. Conference on treatment of phenylketonuria. *J Pediatr* 70(Jan):142-147 (1967).

14. Committee on Fetus and Newborns, American Academy of Pediatrics Statement. *Pediatr* 35:499-500 (1964).

15. Committee on the Handicapped Child, American Academy of Pediatrics Statement on phenylketonuria. *Pediatr* 35:501-503 (1965).

15. Committee on the Handicapped Child, American Academy of Pediatrics. Statement on phenylketonuria. *Pediatr* 35:501-503 (1965).

16. Committee on Nutrition, American Academy of Pediatrics *Report to the Children's Bureau.* (July 30, 1995).

17. Children's Bureau. Minutes of Children's Bureau ad hoc committee on medical genetics. (March 11). File 4-4-1 (1966).

18. G. A. Jervis. The genetics of phenylpyruvic oligophrenia (a contribution to the study of the influence of heredity on mental defect). *Journal of Mental Science* 85:719-62 (1939).

19. L. S. Penrose. *The Influence of Heredity on Disease.* p. 15 (London: H. K. Lewis: 1934).

20. D. J. Kevles. *In the Name of Eugenics: Genetics and the Uses of Human Heredity.* pp. 177-78 (New York: Alfred A. Knopf: 1985).

21. L. I. Woolf and D. G. Vulliamy. Phenylketonuria with a study of the effect upon it of glutamic acid. *Arch Dis Child* 26:487-94.

22. L. I. Woolf, R. Griffiths, and A. Moncrieff. A treatment of phenylketonuria with a diet low in phenylalanine. *Brit Med J.* 1:57-64 (Jan. 8, 1955).

23. H. Bickel, J. Gerard, and E. M. Hickmans. Influence of phenylalanine intake on phenylketonuria. *Lancet* 2(Oct. 17):812-13 (1953).

24. H. Bickel. The effects of a phenylalanine-free and phenylalanine-poor diet in phenylpyruvic oligophrenia. *Experimental Medicine and Surgery* 12:114-18 (1954).

25. H. Bickel. The first treatment of phenylketonuria. *Eur J Pediatr* 155(Suppl 1):S2-S3 (1996).

26. M. D. Armstrong and F. H. Tyler. Studies on phenylketonuria: restricted phenylalanine intake. *J Clin Invest* 34:565-80 (1955).

27. F. Horner and C. Streamer. Effect of phenylalanine-restricted diet on patients with phenylketonuria: clinical observations in three cases. *JAMA* 161:1628-30 (1956).

28. E. A. Knox. An evaluation of the treatment of phenylketonuria with diets low in phenylalanine. *Pediatr* 26:1-11 (1960).

29. H. Bickel and W. Grueter. The dietary treatment of phenylketonuria — experiences during the past 9 years. In: P. J. Bowman and H. V. Mautner. *Mental Retardation: Proceedings of the First International Medical Conference at Portland, Maine.* p. 272 (New York: Grune and Stratton: 1960).

30. B. N. LaDu. The importance of early diagnosis and treatment of phenylketonuria. *Ann Intern Med* 51:1427-33 (1959).

31. W. R. Centerwall, R. F. Chinnock, and A. Pusavat. Phenylketonuria: Screening programs and testing methods. *Am J Public Health* 60:1667-77 (1960).

32. Bickel and Grueter. p. 274 (1960).

33. H. N. Kirkman, Enzyme defects. *Progress in Medical Genetics* 8:125-68 (1972).

34. R. Guthrie. Newborn screening: Past, present and future. Speech presented at Birth Defects Symposium, Albany, NY (Oct. 1, 1985). The copy used here is from the records of the Children's Bureau.

35. R. Guthrie, and A. Susi. A simple phenylalanine method for detecting phenylketonuria in large populations of newborn infants. *Pediatr* 32:338-43 (1963).

36. P. J. Edelson. *History of genetic screening in the United States I: The public debate over phenylketonuria (PKU) testing.* Paper presented at the American Association for the History of Medicine, 1994.

37. R. Brecher and E. Brecher. Saving children from mental retardation. *Saturday Evening Post,* p. 110 (November 21, 1959).

38. P. J. Edelson, *History of genetic screening in the United States I: The public debate over phenylketonuria (PKU) testing.*

39. D. B. Paul and P. J. Edelson, The struggle over metabolic screening. In S. deChaderevian and H. Kamminga, eds. *Molecularising Biology and Medicine:* New practices and alliances, 1930s-1970s: pp. 203-220 (Reading: Harwood Academic Publishers: 1998).

40. Theodore D Tjossem to Arthur J. Lesser. Memo. July 9, 1964.

41. Congressional Record, Senate No. 27919. October 31, 1965.

42. G. A. Jervis. The genetics of phenylpyruvic oligophrenia (a contribution to the study of the influence of heredity on mental defect). *Journal of Mental Science* 85:719-62 (1939).

43. S. S. Rosenberg. A new life for Karen. *Family Weekly* pp. 6-7 (December 16, 1962).

44. L. Pompian. Far-reaching fight against mental retardation. *Today's Health* 39:46, 60-63 (May, 1961) p. 61.

45. Greer p. 25 (1996).

46. National Research Council, Committee for the Study of Inborn Errors of Metabolism. p. 28 (1975).

47. Committee on the Handicapped Child, p. 502 (1965).

48. D. S. Kleinman. Phenylketonuria. A review of some deficits in our information. *Pediatr* 33 (Jan.):125 (1964).

49. S. P. Bessman. Legislation and advances in medical knowledge — acceleration or inhibition? *J Pediatr* 69 (Aug.):334-38 (1966).

50. S. P. Bessman. Implications of the drive for screening. In: J.A. Anderson and K.F. Swaiman, eds. *Phenylketonuria and Allied Metabolic Diseases.* Proceedings of a conference held at Washington, D.C. April 6-8, 1966, (Washington, D.C.: U. S. Government Printing Office: 1967).

51. S. P. Bessman, M. W. Williamson, and R. Koch. Diet, genetics, and mental retardation interaction between phenylketonuric heterozygous mother and fetus to produce nonspecific diminution of IQ: Evidence in support of the justification hypothesis. *Proceedings of the National Academy of Sciences* 75:1562-66 (1978).

52. J. D. Cooper. Problems of legislation in the field of mental retardation. *Rosewood State Hospital Scientific Seminars.* Unpublished paper (Nov. 21, 1965).

53. J. D. Cooper. More problems. *Saturday Review* 50:56-61 (June 3, 1967).

54. Cooper. p. 13 (1965).

55. Edelson. (1994)

56. R. Guthrie. Phenylketonuria detection in the young infant as a routine hospital procedure: A trial of a phenylalanine screening method in 400,000 infants. Children's Bureau unpublished report. (May 2, 1962).

57. R. Guthrie and A. Susi. (1963).

58. Kleinman. p. 124 (1964).

59. Children's Bureau Recommended guidelines for development of PKU screening programs. (Feb. 28) File 4-5-11-5 (1966b).

60. California State Department of Public Health, Bureau of Maternal and Child Health Phenylketonuria and the Guthrie inhibition assay screening procedure. Summary of meeting of consultants to the California State Department of Public Health. *Pediatr* 32(Sept.):345-46 (1963).

61. N. A. Holtzman, A. G. Meek, and E. D. Mellits. Neonatal screening for phenylketonuria: I. Effectiveness. *JAMA* 229(Aug. 5):667-70 (1974).

62. H. M. Nitowsky. Prescriptive screening for inborn errors of metabolism: A critique. *American Journal of Mental Deficiency* 77 (March):539 (1973).

63. Guthrie and Susi. pp. 341-42 (1963).

64. C. C. Mabry, T. L. Nelson and F. A. Horner. Occult phenylketonuria. *Clinical Pediatr* 1:82-86 (1962).

65. J. L. Berman, G. C. Cunningham, R. W. Day, R. Ford, D. Y. Y. Hsia. Causes for high phenylalanine with normal tyrosine in newborn screening programs. *Am J Dis Child* 117:54-65 (1969).

66. M. E. O. Flynn, N. A. Holtzman, M. Blaskovics, C. Azen, M. L. Williamson. The diagnosis of phenylketonuria: A report from the collaborative study of children treated for phenylketonuria. *Am J Dis Child* 134:769-774 (1980).

67. F. Guttler, P. Guldberg, K. F. Henriksen, I. Mikkelsen, B. Olsen, H. Lou. Molecular basis for the phenotypical diversity of phenylketonuria and related hyperphenylalaemias. *J Inherited Metabolic Disease* 16:602-94 (1993).

68. A. Diamond. Phenylalanine levels of 6-10 mg/del may not be as benign as once thought. *Acta Paediatr* 407(Suppl):89-91 (1994).

69. L. I. Woolf. Large-scale screening for metabolic disease in the newborn in Great Britain. In: J. A. Anderson and K. F. Swaiman, eds. Phenylketonuria and Allied Metabolic Disorders. Proceedings of a conference held at Washington, DC, April 6-8, 1966. P. 58 (Washington, DC: U.S. Government Printing Office: 1967).

70. For a wide range of contemporary views, see Anderson and Swaiman pp. 59-61, 113-115 (1967).

71. W. B. Hanley, W. B. Linsao, W. Davison, and C. A. Moes. Malnutrition with early treatment of phenylketonuria. *Pediatric Research* 4:318-327 (1970).

72. F. A. Horner, C. W. Streamer, L. J. Alejandrino, L. H. Reed, and F. Ibbott. Termination of dietary treatment of phenylketonuria. *New J Engl Med* 266:79-81 (1962).

73. R. Koch. Pediatric aspects of phenylketonuria. Children's Bureau, U.S. Dept. of Health, Education and Welfare. (Washington, DC: U.S. Government Printing Office: 1964).

74. H. Bickel and W. Grueter. Management of phenylketonuria. In: F. Lyman, ed., *Management of Phenylketonuria.* pp. 136-72 (Springfield, Il.:Charles Thomas: 1963).

75. Rosenberg. p. 7 (1962).

76. Department of Health, Education, and Welfare, *Mental Retardation Activities of the Department of Health, Education, and Welfare, (March)* p. 3 (Office of Mental Retardation Coordination, Washington, D.C.) 1972.

77. R. A. MacCready. PKU testing: A reply to Professor Cooper. *Medical Tribune* (April 6,1966).

78. Children's Bureau (March 11) p. 4. (1966a).

79. J. P. Swazey. Phenylketonuria: A case study in biomedical legislation. *Journal of Urban Law* 48:923-26 (June 1971).

80. N. A. Holtzman. Anatomy of a Trial. *Pediatrics* 60:932-4 (1977).

81. S. Hellman and D. S. Hellman. Of mice and men: problems of the randomized clinical trial. *N Engl J Med* 324 (May 30):1585-89 (1991).

82. For a recent summary of findings, see C. G. Azen, R. Koch, E. Friedman, E. Wenz, and K. Fishler. Summary of findings from the United States Collaborative Study of children treated for phenylketonuria. *Euro J Pediatr* 155(Suppl 1):S29-S32 (1996).
mmmm 156
89. A. Thompson. Phenylketonuria: An unfolding story. In: M. M. Robertson and V. Eaten, eds. *Movement and Allied Disorders of Childhood* (New York: John Wiley: 1995).

84. S. Waisbren and H. Levy. Agoraphobia in phenylketonuria. *Journal of Inherited Metabolic Disorders* 14:755-64 (1991).

85. J. Weglage, B. Funders, B. Wilken, et al. Psychological and social findings in adolescents with phenylketonuria. *Eur J Pediatr* 151:522-525 (1992).

86. H. L. Levy. Nutritional therapy in inborn errors of metabolism. In: R. J. Desnick, ed. *Treatment of Genetic Diseases.* (New York: Churchill Livingstone: 1991).

87. I. Smith. Treatment of phenylalanine hydroxylase deficiency. *Acta Pediatr* 407 (Suppl):60-65 (1994).

88. S. Waisbren and J. Zaff. Personality disorder in young women with treated phenylketonuria. *Journal of Inherited Metabolic Disorders* 17:584-92 (1994).

89. A. Thompson. Phenylketonuria: An unfolding story. In: M.M. Robertson and V. Eaten, eds. *Movement and Allied Disorders of Childhood* .(New York: John Wiley: 1995).

90. J .Weglage, M. Pietsch, B. Funders, H. G. Koch, and K. Ullrich. Deficits in selective and sustained attention processes in early treated children with phenylketonuria — result of impaired frontal lobe functions? *Eur J Pediatr* 155:200-204 (1996a).

91. J. Weglage, B. Funders, K. Ullrich, A. Rupp, and E. Schmidt. Psychosocial aspects in phenylketonuria. *Eur J Pediatr* 155(Suppl 1):S102-S104 (1996b).

92. V. Schuett. Off-diet young adults with PKU: Lives in danger. *National PKU News* 8(Winter):3 (1997).

93. M. G. Beasley, P. M. Costello, and I. Smith. Outcome of treatment in young adults with phenylketonuria detected by routine neonatal screening between 1964 and 1971. *Quart J Med* 87(Mar):155-160 (1994).

94. D. P. Brenton, A. C. Tarn, J. C. Cabrera-Abreu, and M. Lilburn. Phenylketonuria: treatment in adolescence and adult life. *Eur J Pediatr* 155(Suppl 1):S93-S96 (1996).

95. Medical Research Council. Phenylketonuria due to phenylalanine hydroxylase deficiency: An unfolding story. *Br Med J* 306:115-119 (January 9, 1993).

96. For a review of who pays, see: Illinois Dept of Public Health. Newborn Screening: An Overview of *Newborn Screening Programs in the United States and Canada.* p. 258 (1990).

97. E. W. Clayton. Screening and treatment of newborns. *Houston Law Review* 29:129-30 (1992).

98. B. N. Millner. Insurance coverage of special foods needed in the treatment of phenylketonuria. *Pub Health Rep* 108:64 (1993).

99. D. T. Zallen. *Does it Run in the Family? A Consumer's Guide to DNA Testing for Genetic Disorders.* (New Brunswick, NJ: Rutgers University Press: 1997).

100. Clayon p. 101 (1992).

101. P. G. Kittler and K. Sucher. *Food and Culture in American: A Nutrition Handbook.* pp. 4-5 (New York: Van Nostrand Reinhold: 1989).

102. P. St. James. *The Resource Mothers Program for Maternal PKU: An Ecological Approach to Intervention and Program Evaluation.* p. 101, Ph.D. diss., University of Massachusetts at Boston (1996).

103. M. Douglas. Deciphering a meal. In: *Implicit Meanings: Essays in Anthropology* pp. 249-75 (London and Boston: Routledge and Kegan Paul: 1975). Originally appeared in Daedalus 101:61-81 (1972).

104. Kittler and Sucher. p. 8 (1989).

105. B. J. Anderson. Childhood and adolescent psychological development in relation to diabetes. In: C. Kelnar, ed. *Childhood and Adolescent Diabetes* p. 115 (London: Chapman and Hall: 1995).

106. P. B. Hitchcock, P. J. Brantley, G. N. Jones, G. T. McKnight. Stress and social support as predictors of dietary compliance in hemodialysis patients. *Behavioral Medicine* 18 (Spring:13 (1992).

107. S. E. Waisbren, H. Rokni, I. Bailey, F. Rohr, T. Brown and J. Warner-Rogers. Social factors and the meaning of food in adherence to medical diets: Results of a maternal phenylketonuria summer camp. *Journal of Inherited Metabolic Disorders* 20:21-27 (1997).

108. H. L. Levy and M. Ghavami. Maternal phenylketonuria: A metabolic teratogen. Teratology 53:177 (1996).

109. St. James. p. 99 (1996).

110. C. R. Scriver. The hyperphenylalaninemias of man and mouse. *Annual Review of Genetics* 28:144 (1994).

111. S. E. Waisbren, L. B. Doherty, I. V. Bailey, F. J. Rohr, and H. L. Levy. The New England maternal PKU project: identification of at-risk women. *Am J Public Health* 78:789 (1988).

112. C. G. Azen, R. Koch, E. G. Friedman, *et al.* Intellectual development in 12-year-old children treated for phenylketonuria. *Am J Dis Child* 145:35-39 (1991).

113. R. Koch, H. L. Lelvy, R. Matalon, et al. The international collaborative study of maternal phenylketonuria: Status report 1994. *Acta Paediatrica* 407 (Suppl):112, 113, 118 (1994).

114. E. G. Friedman, R. Koch, C. Azen, *et al.* The international collaborative study on maternal phenylketonuria: Organization, study design and description of the sample. *Eur J Pediatr* 155(Suppl 1):S158-S161 (1996).

115. C. E. Dent. Discussion of Armstrong, M.D.: Relation of biochemical abnormality to development of mental defect in phenylketonuria. In: *Etiologic Factors In Mental Retardation: Report Of Twenty-Third Ross Pediatric Research Conference* (Columbus, Ohio: Ross Laboratories: Nov. 8-9, 1957).

116. C. C. Mabry, T. C. Denniston, T. L. Nelson, and C. D. Son. Maternal phenylketonuria: A cause of mental retardation in children without the metabolic disorder. *New Engl J Med* 269:1404 (Dec. 26, 1963).

117. J. C. Denniston. Children of mothers with phenylketonuria. J. Pediatr 63:461-62 (1963).

118. C. C. Mabry, J. C. Denniston and J. G. Coldwell. Mental retardation in children of phenylketonuric mothers. *New Engl J Med* 275:1331-1336 (Dec. 15,1966).

119. D. Y.-Y Hsia. *Inborn Errors of Metabolism, Part I. Clinical Aspects.* 2nd ed. (Chicago: Year Book Medical Publishers: 1966).

120. J .D. Allan and J. K. Brown. Maternal phenylketonuria and fetal brain damage. In: K.S. Holt and V. P. Coffey. *Some Recent Advances in Inborn Errors of Metabolism* (London: E & S Livingstone: 1968).

121. R. R. Lenke and H. L. Levy. Maternal phenylketonuria and hyperphenylalaninemia: An international survey of the outcome of untreated and treated pregnancies. *New Engl J Med* 303:1202-1208 (Nov. 20,1980).

122. Maternal Phenylketonuria Editorial. *New Engl J Med* 275:1379-80. Dec. 15,1966.

123. P. J. Edelson. Lessons from the history of genetic screening in the US: Policy past, present, and future. In: P. Boyle and K. Nolan, eds. Setting Priorities for Genetic Services (Washington, DC: Georgetown University Press: In press).

124. Ellen S. Kang to Mary Egan, Jan. 4, 1967.

125. National Research Council p. 93 (1975).

126. Nitowsky p. 542 (1973).

127. L. B. Andrews, J. E. Fullarton, N. A. Holtzman, and A. G. Motulsky, eds. *Assessing Genetic Risks: Implications for Health and Social Policy*. Committee on Assessing Genetic Risks, Division of Health Sciences Policy, Institute of Medicine. p. 66 (Washington, D.C.: National Academy Press: 1994).

128. Paul Edelson, personal communication.

129. Medicus Systems Corporation *Cost-Benefit Formulation for Newborn Screening Programs (PKU and Hypothyroidism)*. (July). Prepared under Subcontract to Family Health Care, S.E., Inc. V-2 (1983).

130. For other complications see National Research Council pp. 200-13 (1975).

131. C. R. Scriver. PKU and beyond: When do costs exceed benefits? *Pediatr* 54:617 (1974).

132. U.S. Congress, Office of Technology Assessment, Healthy Children: Investing in the Future. OTA-H-345 pp. 93-116 (Washington, DC: U.S. Government Printing Office: February 1988).

133. L. B. Russell. *Educated Guesses: Making Policy about Medical Screening Tests*. (Berkeley: University of California Press: 1994).

134. S. E. Waisbren, S. Shiloh, P. St. James, and H. L. Levy. Psychosocial factors in maternal phenylketonuria: Prevention of unplanned pregnancies. *Am J Public Health* 81:299-304 (1991).

135. Friedman. p. S160 (1996).

136. H. N. Kirkman. Projections of a rebound in frequency of mental retardation from phenylketonuria. *Applied Research in Mental Retardation* 3:319-28 (1982).

137. N. A. Holtzman. What drives neonatal screening programs? *New Engl J Med* 325(Sept. 12):802-804 (1991).

APPENDIX 6. SCIENTIFIC ADVANCES AND SOCIAL RISKS: HISTORICAL PERSPECTIVES OF GENETIC SCREENING PROGRAMS FOR SICKLE CELL DISEASE, TAY-SACHS DISEASE, NEURAL TUBE DEFECTS AND DOWN SYNDROME, 1970-1997[a]

Howard Markel, M.D., Ph.D.[b]

INTRODUCTION

Scientific research on the genetic basis of human disease has made breathtaking progress over the past several decades, providing an enormous increase in genetic tools for diagnosis, and also posing critical, confounding problems. This essay will historically analyze three genetics testing programs over the past quarter century in order to elucidate some of these problems, and help in developing genetics screening policies that are ethical and effective.

Public assessments of new genetic research have predicted a vast array of diagnostic and therapeutic technologies by the close of the twentieth century.[1,2] Of course it is not possible to forecast just how many pathological conditions will be genetically diagnosed or treated in the next millennium, but physicians, epidemiologists, public health professionals, insurance companies, and patients, to name a few, will have strikingly more genetically based tools available to them. In principal, these tools and the mass screening programs that may be developed from them will facilitate informed reproductive decisions and, when possible, allow physicians to treat and prevent disease.

Exuberance over this progress has been tempered by a growing set of questions: Scientifically, will testing for genetic susceptibility to common complex disorders be sufficiently sensitive, and will it have enough positive predictive value to gain wide acceptance as a predictor of those at risk of future disease? Will these exciting new technologies be sabotaged by the serious medical, psychological, ethical, and legal problems that may be associated with them?[3]

Previous applications of genetic theories to social and public health policies in American history suggest that cultural attitudes toward illness and abnormality run deep. They may force themselves into the debate about how best to apply and interpret genetic screening and therapeutic technologies. There are a number of other issues: race, ethnicity, and gender can affect the understanding of genetic disease; patients, physicians, and genetic counselors must know how to interpret test results; laboratory accuracy and validity data are vital; family members are affected by test outcomes; confidentiality is particularly essential; predictive tests may seriously impact a patient's health and life insurance, and ethical dilemmas arise when the only prevention of some genetic diseases is termination of a pregnancy.

These significant problems may not be considered by the scientist at the laboratory bench or the well-intentioned health care provider who orders a genetic test.

---

[a]The Task Force commissioned this paper and reviewed an early draft of it. The views expressed in this paper are those of the author and do not necessarily reflect the views of the Task Force.

[b]Assistant Professor of Pediatrics and Communicable Diseases, and Director, The Historical Center for the Health Sciences The University of Michigan Medical School, Ann Arbor, Michigan 48109

History is, at best, a less-than-perfect approximation of the present, let alone of the future. But its analysis does provide a means to consider events from earlier genetic screening programs that may have become both culturally embedded and actively present in current social responses. In particular, this essay will discuss the social historical contexts of three applications of genetic screening tools to the diagnosis of disease in the United States during the past quarter century: 1) the Sickle Cell Anemia (SCA) screening programs of the early 1970s; 2) the Tay-Sachs disease (TS) screening programs of the same era; and 3) the maternal alpha-fetoprotein (AFP) prenatal screens for neural tube defects and Down syndrome which began to be mass-marketed during the 1980s.

SICKLE CELL DISEASE AND THE AFRICAN-AMERICAN POPULATION, 1970-1975: THE RELATIONSHIP OF RACE AND GENETIC DISEASE[4]

It is difficult to pinpoint exactly why a collection of public health agencies, physicians, African-American activists, and the Federal and several state governments chose, from all the pressing medical and socioeconomic needs of the African-American community during the early 1970s, to focus on the implementation of mandatory sickle cell screening laws.[5] Even now there is no definitive curative treatment for sickle cell anemia, a disease that affects one out of every 400 to 600 African Americans, or 0.2 percent of that population. (One out of every 10 to 12 African-Americans are carriers of the trait.)

The majority of those screened for sickle cell in the early 1970s were school-aged children or young adults. If any of these individuals actually had sickle cell disease, they probably already had been clinically diagnosed. Because there was no definitive treatment to prevent damage, they were highly likely to have already been harmed. Nor, at that time, was there any safe and inexpensive means of making a prenatal diagnosis of sickle cell anemia in the developing fetus. (It was not until 1978 that Y. W. Kan developed the DNA limited marker test.[6]) Since prenatal diagnosis was virtually not possible, and there were no curative therapies, what did the early sickle cell screening programs hope to accomplish? As Holtzman observed, the "compelling public health interest served by these laws is difficult to discern."[7]

The early 1970s coincided with the peak of the Civil Rights movement, wider voter registration among African Americans, an increase in the number of African-American elected officials, and African-American activism ranging from that of clergy and church-based groups to the Black Panthers.[8,9] In response to the maelstrom of social forces then engulfing the African-American community, President Richard Nixon issued a number of executive orders. A presidential initiative in 1971 increased federal support for the treatment of and research on, sickle cell anemia (approximately $6 million a year). That same year, U.S. Senate hearings on the establishment of a national sickle cell anemia program were initiated. Between 1970 and 1972, twelve states and the District of Columbia enacted mandatory sickle cell screening laws for African-American citizens. More often than not, however, these laws were written and passed without adequate attention to the stigmatizing of not only those people with the disease, but also of those who carried the sickle cell trait. As Reilly concluded in his analysis of the early sickle cell programs: "In retrospect it is clear that the haste with which these laws were drafted and passed contributed substantially to the acrimonious controversy that soon engulfed screening practices."[10]

Several major criticisms of the early sickle cell screening programs have been identified. These criticisms include: 1) a lack of sensitivity to issues of race; 2) controversy surrounding the accuracy and validity of the early screening tests; and 3) inadequate protection of the patient's rights.[11]

Race and Genetics. The most serious criticism of the early sickle cell screening programs has to do with the racial issues surrounding the disease. The initial programs were directed almost exclusively at African-Americans. The briefest review of some of the laws mandating these programs supports that a specific net was cast for African Americans. For example, the New York State law ordered that all persons "not of the Caucasian, Indian, or Oriental races" be tested for sickle cell trait before being allowed to obtain a marriage license. A subsequent New York State law required all urban (but not suburban or rural) schoolchildren to be screened with the tacit understanding that the overwhelming majority of African Americans living in New York at that time were urban dwellers. A similar law enacted in the District of Columbia went one step further in the process of genetic isolation by referring to the blood dyscrasia as a "communicable disease," a term traditionally reserved for infectious rather than inherited diseases and implying the need for quarantine or ostracism.[12,13]

The compulsory screening laws directed at only African Americans obscured the fact that ethnic groups other than blacks can carry the trait and suffer from sickle cell anemia (e.g., people of Mediterranean origins), an omission that ethicist John Fletcher characterized as "racial obfuscation."[14] The national focus on a relatively rare genetic disease presented as "the most vital health issue" facing African Americans also presented several extremely negative political implications—a situation which was not lost on the black community.[15,16] For example, Bryant Rollins, the executive editor of the Amsterdam News (New York City), noted that the federal government's award of a five-year $2.5 million grant to the Harlem Hospital for sickle cell research was far from ideal: "If you read the fine print, there is another side to this grant, the effect of which is to rob the Harlem community of $1 million in much needed funds" that might be better applied to the myriad social, economic, and health problems affecting it.[c]

Misinterpretation of Test Results. A second criticism of the initial sickle cell screening programs was the potential for misinterpretation of the results. At some centers, the validity of the screening methods themselves became the subject of controversy. There were several documented reports of the misuse of the Sickledex test (which does not distinguish trait from homozygous affected) and of the poor quality of many of the laboratories performing the tests, sometimes under state mandates.[17,18] Many of the state and local programs were based on an inadequate knowledge of the genetics of sickle cell disease and as a consequence many of the laws needlessly stigmatized carriers of the sickle cell trait as well as those with the illness. Perhaps most glaring was the apparent ease with which the diagnosis of a heterozygote "carrier status" of sickle cell anemia was used almost interchangeably with homozygote "disease status."

The ostracism of sickle cell carriers, unfortunately, became far more than a theoretical concern for African Americans and public health officials. One especially outrageous diatribe by

---

[c]*Amsterdam News* (New York City) p. 6. (June 1, 1972). The *News* (now the *Amsterdam Star-News*) has long been the leading newspaper of the Harlem, New York City African-American population.

the late scientist and Nobel laureate Linus C. Pauling published in a February, 1968 issue of the UCLA Law Review reflects this stigmatization process of sickle cell carriers: "There should be tattooed on the forehead of every young person, a symbol showing possession of the sickle cell gene [so as to prevent] two young people carrying the same seriously defective gene in single dose from falling in love with one another."[19]

More seriously, by the early 1970s many African Americans were stigmatized by their carrier status in the form of being denied health and life insurance, employment opportunities, and even acceptance into the U.S. Air Force Academy. The African-American community soon perceived the psychosocial risks of the sickle cell screening programs and many persons expressed anger at being further discriminated against for simply being a carrier of sickle cell trait.[20,21]

Inadequate education and counseling at many of the early screening programs only contributed to the milieu of confusion, stigma, and what Abraham Bergman and his colleagues called "sickle cell 'nondisease.'"[d,22] To make matters worse, many American physicians then were not well educated in the diagnosis and management of genetic diseases. For example, in a 1974 survey of 160 physicians' knowledge about sickle cell anemia, one in seven believed sickle cell trait to be indicative of a disease state; one in five found it difficult to clinically distinguish the trait from the disease, and one in two was unaware of the existence of the SC and the S-thal phenotypes.[23]

Some community leaders responded by urging blacks to boycott the sickle cell screening programs. For example, in 1972, Ted Veal, a representative of the African-American activist group, the People's Health Council of New York, described the mandatory screening programs as "genocidal health practices" of the white medical establishment.[24] Indeed, sickle cell screening programs of the early 1970s produced a negative label of disease for an easily identifiable social group that had a long history of being the victims of social discrimination. That made the screening markedly different and far more dangerous in a social context than those programs developed during the same time period for diseases without an ethnic or racial association.[25]

<u>Protection of the Patient's Rights.</u> The third major objection to these early sickle cell screening programs was that in the rush to get the laws into print, many vital protective clauses were omitted, although we have since learned from hard experience to incorporate them. Features that might have tempered the harsh process of genetic stigmatization such as test result confidentiality, competent genetic counseling for people with the trait and the disease, adequate public education on issues of genetic diseases and carrier status, guaranteed medical benefits for those afflicted with sickle cell anemia, and uniform guidelines to ensure quality control of the testing and laboratory facilities were either not considered or were patently ignored by those drafting the original sickle cell legislation.[26, 27]

The problems of this particular application of genetics to social policy began to be recognized soon after the enactment of the state laws described above. By late 1972, Congress passed the National Sickle Cell Anemia Control Act, which reflected a number of these concerns. Although these problems were not rectified immediately, the energetic efforts of the African-American and medical communities, in addition to numerous legislators, lawyers, and public policymakers, helped to modify and greatly improve use of sickle cell anemia screening technologies. For example, during the 1980s, it was found that newborn screening for sickle cell anemia was justified because of the

---

[d]These investigators recommended against mass screening of children for sickle cell disease although they agreed with the selective use of prenatal diagnosis for sickle cell trait in prospective parents.

ability of antibiotics to prevent serious and sometimes fatal infections in children with sickle cell anemia.[28] In addition, newly developed pneumococcal vaccines have contributed to the reduction of early death due to susceptibility to pneumococcal infections. Many African-American parents recognized the value of the sickle cell newborn screen. Still, some clinicians continue to find evidence of fear and avoidance of all forms of sickle cell testing especially among those African-Americans with relatives who underwent testing during the 1970s.[29] In a study conducted in Rochester, New York during the 1980s, less than half of the pregnant African-American women at risk of having affected fetuses utilized prenatal diagnosis technologies.[30]

TAY-SACHS DISEASE AND THE ASHKENAZI JEWISH-AMERICAN COMMUNITY, 1970-1980: THE IMPORTANCE OF INCLUDING THE COMMUNITY IN SCREENING PROGRAMS

Genetic screening for Tay-Sachs disease began to be developed about the same time as the early sickle cell screening programs discussed above. Like sickle cell disease, Tay-Sachs was found to occur predominantly in one defined ethnic population—infants of Ashkenazi (East European) Jewish ancestry. Unlike sickle cell disease, however, which can vary greatly in clinical symptoms and severity from patient to patient, Tay-Sachs victims had no hope of productive life and faced irreversible and progressive neurodegeneration, dementia, and death during the first five years of life.[31,32,33] Indeed, given the state of the art in medical care for Tay-Sachs disease during this period, the soundest public health approach to the problem was avoiding the birth of the affected fetus. Ashkenazi Jews and African Americans had very different experiences with their genetic testing.[34] In the first place, the reproductive choices for Tay-Sachs disease were less ambiguous when compared to sickle cell anemia; prenatal diagnosis for Tay-Sachs was possible.[35,36,37] Then, too, there were striking social differences between them. The Jewish-American community was no stranger to discrimination, particularly in its relation to the application of genetic theory to social policy. Many of those enrolling in the Tay-Sachs screening programs of the 1970s were, literally, the grandchildren of the East European Jewish immigrants who were stigmatized during the 1920s and accused of importing inferior genes and "protoplasm" into the United States.[38,39,40] Yet with the passage of time and acquisition of the confidence of assimilation, Jewish-Americans of the 1970s generally expressed fewer fears of discrimination than their African-American counterparts when confronted with these new screening technologies. There were some, however, who did not support Tay-Sachs screening.[41,42]

This difference of perception may have been due to the social experiences of these two ethnic groups in the United States over the past two centuries. By the early 1970s, the lives of Jewish-Americans (both those originating from Germany and Eastern Europe) had, for the most part, markedly improved by all economic and social markers. Members of the African-American community, on the other hand, remained the target for a number of forms of discrimination and were actively fighting for basic civil rights. The latter group was particularly vulnerable to additional stigmatization in the form of a genetic label and less likely to view government or institutional involvement in health assessment as a positive development.

It is important that while the early Tay-Sachs programs were not extensively taken up by the entire Jewish-American community, many of their innovative features were subsequently found to be of great value. The same approach was used 25 years later to organize a study of heritable breast cancer in Ashkenazi Jews.[43] Some of the earliest Tay-Sachs programs were organized at synagogues. In advance of implementing the screening programs, a series of productive meetings and discussion forums were held between physicians, ethicists, rabbis, and other members of the particular Jewish religious communities. As a result of these meetings, physicians and public health workers developed programs that focused on young Ashkenazi Jewish married couples who were considering having a child; other programs expanded this target group to include all unmarried members of the Ashkenazi Jewish community who were 18 years old or older.

Another positive feature of the early synagogue-based Tay-Sachs screening programs is that religious leaders and community volunteers worked side by side with physicians and genetics counselors to provide education at the screening site as well as to answer any questions the participants might have. Informed consents were routinely obtained and several steps were taken to ensure confidentiality. Those who tested positive for the carrier state were telephoned. Genetic counseling for individuals positive for Tay-Sachs was then offered, especially to those couples who both tested positive for the carrier state. In general, the woman in such couples underwent prenatal diagnostic testing of amniotic fluid when she became pregnant. The majority of those couples who were discovered to be carrying a fetus afflicted with Tay-Sachs disease elected to terminate the pregnancy.[44,45,46,47,48]

This focus on religious institutions and communities was not entirely successful. Not all Jews were members of a synagogue and different areas in the United States and Canada embraced these programs at markedly different rates. For example, in Toronto, the Jewish community actively joined forces with the medical and public health communities to establish programs in the early 1970s, while in Montreal, the Jewish community did not. One impetus for the design of a well-known study was the lack of interest in Tay-Sachs screening among the Montreal Jewish community, leading the investigators to develop a study that "captured" Jewish high school students.[49]

There are, of course, many different sectors of the Jewish-American community, divided along lines of religiosity (e.g., the Orthodox, Conservative, Reform movements, as well as non-practicing or secular Jews), place of geographic origin, economic status, and a number of other social factors that were recognized by the partnership of religious and community leaders and the medical establishment. One effort to address these differences was the Chevra Dor Yeshorim Program of New York City, designed to accommodate the cultural customs and religious beliefs of ultra-Orthodox Jews. Developed in partnership with members of the Orthodox-Hassidic Jewish community, which has a high risk of Tay-Sachs disease and strong opposition to abortion and contraception, this program relies on this community's practice of arranged marriages. When a Hassidic Jewish woman reaches 18 years of age or a man 20, the subject undergoes a blood test for Tay-Sachs disease. The laboratory handling the test assigns a code number to the sample and it is tested anonymously. The results are listed and stored by code number indefinitely. The subject is given only the code number but not the actual results of the test. At the time of a planned marriage, the shadchen, or matchmaker, is given the code numbers of the prospective bride and groom and presents them to the laboratory registry. If both partners are positive for the carrier state, the matchmaker is told that the match is not a good one and another match is arranged. If a couple does not use a matchmaker, they, too, may inquire of their status from the registry and make their decisions accordingly.[e] A central aim of this plan is to keep the effects of genetic stigmatization to a minimum. Couples screening programs have been applied to cystic fibrosis (CF) in Scotland and England, and in Maine. The CF programs are similar to Chevra Dor Yeshorim in that only couples who were both positive for the trait are informed of the result; if only one partner is a carrier, s/he is not informed. The difference is that married couples are tested for CF.[50,51] This program has since been applied to Orthodox Jewish communities elsewhere in the United States, Canada, Europe, and Israel.[52,53]

As large populations were tested, problems surfaced concerning the reliability and validity of the available Tay-Sachs screening tools. For example, the earliest Tay-Sachs screening tests were plagued with an unacceptable rate of "false positives." Women concurrently using oral birth control pills were 50 percent or more likely to have a false-positive carrier test result. Other medications were discovered to be the cause of a false-negative carrier result. Fortunately, several research consortiums that were devoted to the prevention of Tay-Sachs disease conducted follow-up studies to identify and correct such problems in test validity.

The critically important, and potentially overlooked, lesson is that any genetic screening program must provide unrelenting vigilance in the implementation of such tests on large numbers of people, in addition to the careful surveillance of test development.[54]

Since 1971, screening programs directed at the Ashkenazi Jewish population in the United States and Canada have led to a 90 percent reduction in Tay-Sachs disease.[55] The Tay-Sachs screening programs are often recalled as a success in the blending of science, bioethics, and disease prevention. At the same time, several follow-up studies have documented that, although genetic counseling alleviated some of the anxieties experienced by the heterozygous, phenotypically normal Tay-Sachs carriers, there was evidence of residual unease among many of them simply at potentially being labeled a carrier.[56,57,58,59,60]

PRENATAL SCREENS FOR DOWN SYNDROME AND NEURAL TUBE DEFECTS: APPLYING WHAT WE HAVE LEARNED TO THE DEVELOPMENT OF NEW GENETIC SCREENING TESTS

Over the past three decades, a number of technologies have been developed giving physicians better means of gaining information about genetic and physical aspects of the developing fetus. A striking example is Brock and Sutcliffe's 1972 description of the association of elevated levels of amniotic fluid alpha-fetoprotein in the antenatal diagnosis of neural tube defects such as anencephaly and spina bifida.[61] Subsequent studies found an association between elevated maternal serum alpha-fetoprotein (MSAFP) levels and the incidence of neural tube defects.[62]

The transfer of this technology across the Atlantic Ocean might be best characterized as stormy. Early on, several enterprising American biotechnology firms vied to secure the FDA license for the manufacture of AFP screening kits. Initially such distinguished medical bodies as the American College of Obstetrics and Gynecology and the American Academy of Pediatrics, however, expressed serious concerns about the marketing of such a diagnostic tool, given that practicing

---

[e]*Shadchen* is the Yiddish word for matchmaker; *shiddach* is the Hebrew equivalent. Not all of the programs agreed with this set-up. For example, the early Tay-Sachs screening programs in Baltimore, MD strongly discouraged unmarried individuals from testing so as to <u>not</u> influence one's choice of mate among those for whom prenatal diagnosis and abortion were acceptable options.

obstetricians at that time did not fully understand the limitations of the test and the need for follow-up testing.[63] Others wondered if the fragmented, almost cottage-industry American health care system of the early 1980s might create obstructions to conducting a safe and smooth testing program in comparison to the nationalized health care system that existed concurrently in Great Britain.[64]

Politics, too, had a significant effect on these programs, in that the FDA suggested restrictions to the use of AFP kits in 1980 that would have increased the likelihood of a well-run genetics screening program. They were ignored by the Reagan Administration. In spite of the tremendous controversy generated in the United States, the Food and Drug Administration gave pre-market approval to manufacturers of AFP kits in 1983.[65] Soon thereafter, it became fairly routine for physicians to obtain serum alpha-fetoprotein levels of pregnant women in the United States as a screening test for these birth defects.[66]

During the mid-1980s, concurrent work by several geneticists noted the association of low maternal serum alpha-fetoprotein levels with chromosomal abnormalities such as Down syndrome (Trisomy 21) and Trisomy 18.[67,68] The risk of a baby being born with Down syndrome increases with maternal age, and this association is noted in mothers of all ages. For example, while the overall incidence rate for Down syndrome is 1/600-800 live births, the risk of Down syndrome increases with maternal age is markedly more common in a child born to a woman over 35 years of age (1/365), and the rate of incidence increases with each year of age. (e.g., 24-year-old women have an incidence of only 1/1,300, while 40-year-old women have a 1/110 incidence and 45-year-old women have a 1/41 incidence).[69] It is important to note that despite the much higher rate of Down syndrome in the offspring of older pregnant women, the majority of Down syndrome infants are born to younger women, simply because most pregnancies occur in women under 35 years of age. The AFP tests offered a safe, inexpensive (when compared to amniocentesis and karyotyping) means of screening lower-risk younger women who parented the largest number of affected infants. The tests' use has broadened over the past decade and they are routinely offered to those pregnant women who have access to prenatal care in the United States.

The maternal serum alpha-fetoprotein assay is a first-step screening test. It does not diagnose disease; rather it identifies most of those who are deemed to be at increased risk and who require further testing for a definitive diagnosis. A particular benefit to this screening test is that it is a relatively low risk and inexpensive medical procedure. A blood sample is taken from the mother at 15 to 20 weeks of gestation. The recently developed Down syndrome "triple marker" screen of MSAFP, maternal serum unesterified estriol, and maternal serum human chorionic gonadotropin increases the detection rate from 20 percent for MSAFP alone to 60 percent.[70] Elevated or decreased levels are then followed by more definitive, and costly, ultrasonic examination and amniocentesis.[71] It is, therefore, essential for both the health provider and the patient to understand that an elevated AFP is not diagnostic for neural tube defects; nor is a low AFP diagnostic of Down syndrome. These aberrant levels, in fact, may be associated with a large number of disorders or may not be associated with any fetal abnormality at all.[72] There also exists a high association of falsely elevated AFP levels due to misdating of the pregnancy, multiple births, errors in reporting or determining race, diabetes mellitus, errors in calculating body weight, laboratory errors and physician misinterpretation.

Subsequent studies on the interactions between female patient and male health care provider suggest that gender differences have an impact on the patient's own ethical decision making. Wertz has documented how health care providers and patients have significantly different perceptions on the assessment of genetic risks.[73] Press and Browner analyzed the decisions of an ethnically and socioeconomically diverse group of women to refuse or accept a prenatal diagnostic test. The factors that determined the decisionmaking process of these women in the early 1990s was neither ethnic nor social class related; instead, the determining factor was how the women were informed about the tests. Press and Browner hypothesized that the women and health care professionals involved in these clinical interactions create a "collective fiction" that "situate[s] the testing within the domain of routine prenatal care and denie[s] its central connection to selective abortion and its eugenic implications." As a result of these and similar studies of patients' experience undergoing genetic screening tests, we are beginning to appreciate the great potential that exists for patient (and physician) misunderstanding, conflicts over ethnic and gender issues, and anxiety about the test results.[74,75,76,77]

Interestingly, despite close scrutiny by the scientific genetics community, the AFP, estriol, and chorionic gonadotropin ("triple") screens for Down syndrome have not been fully evaluated or regulated by the Food and Drug Administration. A close follow-up of these screens and definitive policies for their use is an important aspect of this program that has not been fully addressed.

CONCLUSIONS

This brief historical review of the sickle cell, Tay-Sachs, neural tube defects and Down syndrome screening programs presents many lessons that can be learned from the past:

• Sensitivity to the needs of the groups screened and the inclusion of those groups in the planning of screening programs can frame the diagnosis and understanding of genetic disease with respect to issues of race, ethnicity, and gender;

• Patients, physicians, and genetic counselors must understand what these tests actually predict or diagnose in order to ensure that patients make fully informed, autonomous decisions about the test results;

• Unrelenting vigilance is necessary on the validity of tests and the reliability of the laboratories providing them, both as the tests are developed and as they are used on large numbers of people;

• It is important to consider how these test results may effect other family members;

• Confidentiality of the information discovered is vital;

• The impact of a genetic diagnosis on the patient's health or life insurance status must be carefully considered; and

• An ethical dilemma is posed by disease avoidance using pregnancy termination.

This last dilemma exemplifies the deeper question of just what one is going to do with the results of these screens. No definitive treatments yet exist for Down syndrome, neural tube defects,

Tay-Sachs disease and many other prenatally detectable genetic conditions. The principal means of disease prevention for these disorders is pregnancy termination.[f]

There are prospective parents for whom abortion is not an acceptable alternative. Early 20th century eugenicists might call such a selection process negative eugenics[g][78]; late 20th century fundamentalist Christians would deem such an option as murder of an unborn child. Similarly, ultra-orthodox Jews and observant Roman Catholics do not accept abortion as an option. Indeed, the health care provider's own views on abortion may have an impact on the information and options provided to the parents of an affected fetus. Furthermore, anti-abortion (pro-life) activists, and their pro-choice or abortion rights counterparts, have become increasingly focused on genetic screening programs since the mid-1980s, which brings a high-stakes political element to the clinical arena.[79] All of these political spins will have to be taken into account as policymakers continue to plan and develop prenatal screening programs for serious diseases that at the present have no treatment.

The benefits and the liabilities of these nascent technologies and medical breakthroughs are of concern to all of society, but are of particularly critical importance to those involved in genetic research, medical practice, and public health policy. New developments will bring both old and new dilemmas to the surface so that some of these issues may become irrelevant, depending on how technology, society, and culture evolve. Other issues, particularly race, ethnicity, and gender, appear to return perennially to genetic testing programs.

If history teaches us anything about genetic screening, and more broadly, about the ethical use of biotechnology, it is that careful discussion and planning goes a long way in ameliorating many of their associated difficult issues. We must address such issues before inappropriate uses or applications become socially embedded in our medical practices and must be open to the recognition of dilemmas that become apparent after the implementation of a genetic screening program.

ABOUT THE AUTHOR

Dr. Markel is Assistant Professsor of Pediatrics and Communicable Diseases and Director of the Historical Center at the University of Michigan. He is a Generalist Physician Faculty Scholar of the Robert Wood Johnson Foundation and a recipient of the James A. Shannon Director's Award of the National Institutes of Health, and the Burroughs-Wellcome History of Medicine Scholars Award. The opinions discussed in this paper are his own and do not necessarily reflect those of the University of Michigan, the Robert Wood Johnson Foundation, the National Institutes of Health, or the Burroughs-Wellcome Foundation.

---

[f] I use the word "principal" rather than "only" decidedly; there are a number of research strategies being developed to avoid the conception of affected fetuses instead of the termination of pregnancies. For example, it has recently found that the maternal intake of folate periconceptionally does reduce the occurrence of neural tube defects; as a result, bread products will soon be required to be supplemented with folate.

[g] Eugenicists defined negative eugenics as the discouragement of the so-called "inferior" or diseased classes from reproducing, including those individuals and social groups believed to be carriers of deleterious traits.

REFERENCES

1. J. D. Watson. The Human Genome Project: past, present, and future, *Science* 248:49-51 (1990).

2. F. Collins and D. Galas. A new five year plan for the U.S. Human Genome Project. *Science* 262:43-46 (1993).

3. L. B. Andrews, J. E. Fullarton, N. A. Holtzman, A. G. Motulsky, eds. *Assessing Genetic Risks: Implications for Health and Social Policy*. (Washington D.C.: National Academy Press: 1994).

4. This section is largely drawn from my longer essay on sickle cell screening programs during the 1970s: H Markel. The stigma of disease: implications of genetic screening. *Am J Med* 93:209-215 (1992).

5. P. Reilly. State supported mass genetic screening programs. In: A. Milunsky, G. J. Annas, eds. pp. 159-184 *Genetics and the Law* (New York: Plenum Press: 1975).

6. Y. W. Kan. Antenatal diagnosis of sickle-cell anemia by DNA analysis of amniotic-fluid cells. *Lancet* ii:910-912 (1978).

7. N. A. Holtzman. *Proceed with caution. Predicting genetic risks in the recombinant DNA era.* p. 219 (Baltimore: Johns Hopkins University Press: 1989).

8. C. F. Whitten. Sickle cell programming: an imperiled promise. *New Engl J Med* 288:318-319 (1973).

9. E. Buetler, D. R. Boggs, P. Heller, *et al.* Hazards of indiscriminate screening for sickling. *New Engl J Med* 285:1485-1486 (1971).

10. P. Reilly. p. 173 (1975).

11. P. Reilly. *Genetics, Law and Social Policy* pp. 67-68 (Cambridge, MA: Harvard University Press: 1977).

12. P. Reilly. Sickle cell anemia legislation. *J Legal Med* 1:36 (1973).

13. M. L. Miringoff. *The Social Costs of Genetic Welfare* p. 50 (New Brunswick, N.J.: Rutgers University Press: 1991).

14. J. Fletcher. Genetics, choice and society. In: N. Lipkin, P.T. Ronley, eds. *Genetic Responsibility: On Choosing Our Children's Genes* p. 95 (New York: Plenum: 1974).

15. D. Wilkinson. For whose benefit? Politics and sickle cell. *The Black Scholar* 5(8):29 (1974).

16. T. Powledge. The new ghetto hustle. *Saturday Review of the Sciences* 569:38-40 (Jan. 27, 1973).

17. U.S. Dept. of Health, Education and Welfare, Public Health Service. *Hemoglobinopathy III: Proficiency Testing, June 1975.* (Atlanta, Ga: Center for Disease Control: 1975).

18. Letter from N A. Holtzman to author, November 12, 1996, in author's possession, used with permission.

19. L. Pauling. Reflections on the new biology. *UCLA Law Review* 15:268-272 (1968).

20. J. Bowman. Invited editorial: prenatal screening for hemoglobinopathies. *Am J Hum Genet* 48:433-438 (1991).

21. B. S. Wilfond, N. Fost. The cystic fibrosis gene: medical and social implications for heterozygote detection. *JAMA* 263:2777-2783 (1990).

22. M. L. Hampton, J. Anderson, B. S. Lavizzo, A. B. Bergman. Sickle cell "nondisease": a potentially serious public health problem. *Am J Dis Child* 128:58-61 (1974).

23. D B. Kellon, E. Buetler. Physician attitudes about sickle cell disease and sickle cell trait. *JAMA* 227:71-72 (1974).

24. *Amsterdam News* (New York City) p 4 (March 18, 1972).

25. Committee for the Study of Inborn Errors of Metabolism, Division of Medical Sciences, Assembly of Life Sciences, National Research Council Barton Childs, ed. *Genetic Screening: Programs, Principles and Research.* pp. 120-127 (Washington D.C.: National Academy of Sciences: 1975).

26. P. Reilly. pp. 172-173 (1975).

27. N. Fost, M. M. Kaback. Why do sickle cell screening in children? The trait is the issue. *Pediatrics* 51:742-745 (1973).

28. M. H. Gaston, J. I Verter, G. Woods, C. Pegelow, J. Kelleher, G. Presbury, E. Zarkowksy, *et al.* Prophylaxis with oral penicillin in Children with sickle cell anemia. *N Engl J Med* 314:1593-9 (1986).

29. Comment of Task Force member cited in a letter from N A. Holtzman to author, November 12, 1996, in author's possession, used with permission.

30. P. T. Rowley, S. Loader, C. J. Sutera, M. Walden, A. Kozyra. Prenatal screening for hemoglobinapathies. I. A prospective regional trial. *Am J Hum Genet* 48:439-446 (1991).

31. M. M. Kaback, J. Lim-Steele, D. Dalholkar, D. Brown, N. Levy, and K. Ziegler. Tay-Sachs disease: carrier screening, prenatal disease, and the molecular era. An international perspective. *JAMA* 270:2307-2315 (1993).

32. W. Tay. Symmetrical changes in the region of the yellow spot in each eye of an infant. *Trans Ophthalm Soc of the United Kingdom* 1:55-57 (1881).

33. B. Sachs. On arrested cerebral development, with special reference to its cortical pathology. *J Nervous and Mental Diseases* 14:541-553 (1887).

34. L. Roberts. To test or not to test. One worked, the other didn't. Tay-sachs disease and sickle cell disease. *Science* 247:17-19 (1990).

35. M. Kaback, R. S. Ziegler. The John F. Kennedy Institute program. Practical and ethical issues in an adult screening program. In: B. Hilton, ed. *Ethical Issues in Genetics: Genetics Counseling and the Use of Genetic Knowledge.* p. 131(New York: Plenum: 1973).

36. The President's Commission for the Study of Ethical Problems in Medicine and Biomedical and Behavioral Research *Screening and Counseling for Genetic Conditions: A Report on the Ethical, Social, and Legal Implications of Genetic Screening, Counseling and Education Programs.* pp. 17-23 (Washington D.C.: Government Printing Office: 1983).

37. Committee for the Study of Inborn Errors of Metabolism pp. 129-132 (1975).

38. H. Markel. *Di goldene Medina* (The golden land): Historical perspectives of eugenics and the east European (Ashkenazi) Jewish-American community, 1880-1925. *Health Matrix: Journal of Law and Medicine* 7(1):49-64 (1997).

39. C. E. Rosenberg. Charles Benedict Davenport and the irony of American eugenics. In: C. E. Rosenberg. *No Other Gods: On Science and American Social Thought* p. 91 (Baltimore: Johns Hopkins University Press: 1976).

40. K. M. Ludmerer. *Genetics and American Society: A Historical Appraisal* pp. 87-119 (Baltimore: Johns Hopkins University Press: 1972).

41. M. J. Goodman, L. E. Goodman. The overselling of genetic anxiety. *Hastings Center Report* 12(5)(Oct.):20-7 (1982).

42. F. Rosner and M. W. Steele. Mass screening for Tay-Sachs disease.*Hastings Center Report* 13(3)(June):44-5 (1983).

43. J. P. Streuwing, P. Hartge, S. Wacholder, S. M. Baker, M. Berlin, M. McAdams, M. M. Timmerman, L. C. Brody and M. A. Tucker. The risk of cancer associated with specific mutations of BRCA1 and BRCA2 among Ashkenazi Jews. *New Eng J Med* 336:1401-8 (1997).

44. *Assessing Genetic Risks* pp 42-43 (1994).

45. M. Kaback, ed. *Tay-Sachs disease: screening and prevention. Proceedings of the first international conference on Tay-Sachs disease* pp. 79-94, 355-366 (New York: Alan R. Liss: 1977).

46. M. M. Kaback, R. S. Zeiger, L. W. Reynolds, M. Sonneborn. Approaches to the control and prevention of Tay-Sachs diseases. *Progress in Medical Genetics* 10:103-134 (1974).

47. F. Massarik, M. M. Kaback, S. Greenwald, T. J. Nathan, M. Rosenthal, D. M. Bass. Community-based genetic education, communication channels, and knowledge of Tay-Sachs disease. *Prog Clin Biol Res* 18:353-366 (1977).

48. M. Kaback, J. Lim-Steele, D. Dabholkar, D. Brown, N. Levy and K. Zeiger. Tay-Sachs disease--carrier screening, prenatal diagnosis, and the molecular era. An international perspective, 1970 to 1993. *JAMA* 270(19):2307-15 (1993).

49. S. Zeeman, C. L. Clow, L. Cartier, C. R. Scriver. A private view of heterozygosity: eight year follow-up on carriers of the Tay-Sachs gene detected by high school screening in Montreal. *Am J Hum Genet* 18:769-778 (1984).

50. N. J. Wald. Couple screening for cystic fibrosis. *Lancet* 338:1318-1319 (1991).

51. R. A. Doherty, G. E. Palamaki, E. M. Kloza, J. L. Erickson, J. E. Haddow. Couple-based prenatal screening for cystic fibrosis in primary care settings. *Prenatal Diagn* 16(5):397-404 (1996).

52. B. Merz. Matchmaking scheme solves Tay-Sachs problem. *JAMA* 258:2636-2639 (1987).

53. B. Childs, L. Gordis, M. M. Kaback, H. H. Kazazian. Tay-Sachs screening: motives for participating and knowledge of genetics and probability. *Am J Hum Genet* 28:537-549 (1976).

54. Letter from M. M. Kaback to N. A. Holtzman, October 21, 1996, in author's possession, used with permission.

55. *Assessing Genetic Risks* p. 43 (1994).

56. B. Childs, L. Gordis, M. M. Kaback, and H. Kazazian. Tay-Sachs screening: social and psychological impact. *Am J Hum Genet* 28:550-558 (1976).

57. B. Childs, L. Gordis, M. M. Kaback, and H. Kazazian. Tay-Sachs screening: motives for participating and knowledge of genetics and probability. *Am J Hum Genet* 28:537-549 (1976).

58. S. Zeeman, E. L. Clow, L. Cartier, C. R. Scriver. A private view of heterozygosity: eight year

mmmm 174

59. F. Rosner. Screening for Tay-Sachs disease: a note of caution. *J Clin Ethics* 2:251-252 (1991).

60. J. J. Mitchell, A. Capua, C. Clow, C. R. Scriver. Twenty-year outcome analysis of genetic screening programs for Tay-Sachs and beta-thalassemia disease carriers in high schools. *Am J Hum Genet* 59(4):793-8 (1996).

61. D. Brock, R. Sutcliffe. Alpha-fetoprotein in the antenatal diagnosis of anencephaly and spina bifida. *Lancet* ii:197 (1972).

62. Report of the U K. Collaborative Study on Alpha-fetoprotein in relation to neural-tube defects: Maternal serum alpha-fetoprotein measurement in antenatal screening for anencephaly and spina bifida in each pregnancy. *Lancet* 1:1324 (1977).

63. N. A. Holtzman. Prenatal Screening for Neural Tube Defects. *Pediatrics* 71:657-659 (1983).

64. N. A. Holtzman. From Research to Routine: How is the Road Paved? In: B. Gastel, J. E. Haddow, J. C. Fletcher, A. Neale, eds. *Maternal Serum Alpha-fetoprotein: Issues in the Prenatal Screening and Diagnosis of Neural Tube Defects.* Proceedings of a conference held by the National Center for Health Care Technology and the Food and Drug Administration. pp. 153-158 (Washington D.C.: July 28-30, 1980).

65. Department of Health and Human Services, Food and Drug Administration Alpha-Fetoprotein kits; withdrawal of proposed rule. *Federal Register* 48:277780-3 (1983).

66. J. D. Davis. Reproductive technologies for prenatal diagnosis. *Fetal Diagn Ther* 8:(Suppl 1):28-38 (1993).

67. I. R. Merkatz, H. M. Nitowsky, J. N. Macri, W. E. Johnson. An association between low maternal serum alpha-fetoprotein and fetal chromosomal abnormalities. *Am J Obstet Gynecol* 184:896 (1984).

68. H. S. Cuckle, N. J. Wald, R. H. Lindenbaum. Maternal serum alpha-fetoprotein measurement: a screening test for Down syndrome. *Lancet* 2:926-929 1984.

69. E. B. Hook, G. M. Chambers. Estimated rates of Down syndrome in live births by one year maternal age intervals of mothers aged 20-49. IN: D. Bergsma, R.B. Lowry, eds. *Numerical Taxonomy of Birth Defects and Polygenic Disorders* p. 126 (New York: Alan R. Liss/March of Dimes Foundation: 1977).

70. J. E. Haddow, G. E. Palomaki, G. J. Knight, *et al.* Prenatal screening for Down's syndrome with use of maternal serum markers. *New Engl J Med* 327:588-593 (1992).

71. *Assessing Genetic Risks* pp. 79-80 (1994).

72. B. K. Burton. Maternal serum alpha feto-protein. *Pediatr Ann* 687-697 (1989).

73. D. C. Wertz. Provider biases and choices: the role of gender. *Clin Obst Gyn* 36:521-531 (1993).

74. N. A. Press, C. H. Browner. 'Collective fictions': similarities in reasons for accepting maternal serum alpha-fetoprotein screening among women of diverse ethnic and social backgrounds. *Fetal Diagn Ther* 8(Suppl. I): 97-106 (1993).

75. R. R. Faden, J. Chadlow, E. Orel-Crosby, *et al.* What participants understand about a maternal serum alpha-fetoprotein screening program. *Am J Pub Health* 75:1381-1384 (1982).

76. A. Lippmann. Prenatal genetic testing and geneticization: mother matters for all. *Fetal Diagn Ther* 8(Suppl. 1):175-188 (1993).

77. D. C. Wertz, J. C. Fletcher. Feminist criticism of prenatal diagnosis: a response. *Clin Obst Gyn* 36:541-567 (1993).

78. D. Kevles. *In the Name of Eugenics. Genetics and the Uses of Human Heredity* p. 85 (New York: Alfred Knopf: 1985).

79. S. D. Lavine. Who deserves to be born: moral implications of genetic testing of fetuses to ensure healthy babies. *New York Times* p. A11 (December 29, 1995).

GLOSSARY

Allele — The actual nucleotide sequence of a gene on a chromosome. Changes in sequence from one allele to another arise as a result of mutation in the germline and can be transmitted to the next generation.

Allelic diversity — Within populations, the presence of different alleles at a gene locus.

Amino acids — The building blocks of proteins. In vertebrates, there are 20 amino acids. In a gene, each amino acid is encoded by a sequence of 3 nucleotides (triplet) that instructs the cell to insert that amino acid in a specific position as the protein is assembled. No triplet encodes for more than one amino acid but different triplets encode for the same amino acid.

Analyte — The substance measured by a laboratory test, for instance, a specific mutation or allele.

Analytical sensitivity, specificity — See Sensitivity, Specificity

Anonymization — Removing all identifiers from a specimen without retaining any code. Consequently, there is no way the specimen can be traced back to the person from which it came.

Autosomal — A gene (or its alleles) on one of the 22 autosomes. See Chromosome

Blind testing — Use of a specimen whose contents are unknown to the laboratory, or to the laboratory technician, to assess the ability of the laboratory to perform a test correctly. Usually the technician is aware that the specimen is being used for quality assessment but does not know (i.e., is blind to) its contents. In the most rigorous blinding, the specimen arrives at the laboratory as a routine specimen.

Carrier — (1) A person of either gender who has inherited a disease-causing autosomal allele from one parent and a normal allele from the other parent. Inheritants of disease-causing alleles from both parents results in an autosomal recessive disease. (2) A female who possesses an allele on one of her X chromosomes (X-linked) which results in disease in males. In most cases, carriers suffer no ill effects from possession of the allele. "Heterozygote" for autosomal recessive or X-linked disorders is a synonym for "carrier." (3) A person who has inherited a single allele which results in an autosomal dominant disease.

Chromosome — The rod-like nucleoproteins along which the genes are arrayed in the nucleus. In human somatic cells, the chromosomes consist of 22 pairs of autosomes and, in females, two X chromosomes and, in males an X chromosome and a Y chromosome. Normally, therefore, each cell contains 46 chromosomes.

Clinical sensitivity, specificity — See Sensitivity, Specificity

DNA — Deoxyribonucleic acid. A linear sequence of deoxyribonucleotides (nucleotides for short). See Nucleotide.

Dominant — A condition that is manifest in heterozygotes.

Enzyme — A protein with a catalytic function (i.e., one that accelerates a chemical reaction reaching equilibrium).

Gene, gene locus — The position on a chromosome at which alleles reside. Alleles are transcribed into mRNA.

Gene product — The mRNA or protein encoded by a specific gene, or more properly, alleles of the gene.

Genetic heterogeneity — (1) The presence of different alleles at a gene locus. See Allelic diversity. (2) The ability of more than one allele to cause the same trait, for instance, a disease. Alleles at different gene loci (locus heterogeneity), as well as those at the same locus (allelic diversity), may each be expressed as the same trait.

Genetic predisposition or susceptibility — A genotype that increases the risk of disease but does not make it certain. The susceptibility-conferring allele will be inherited in Mendelian fashion but the disease itself will not. The single locus genotype is insufficient to result in disease. Impaired expression of alleles at other gene loci and/or environmental factors are needed before disease appears.

Genome — The entire array of genes of an organism or species.

Genotype — (1) The alleles that an individual possesses at a gene locus. One of these alleles is inherited from the mother, the other from the father. (2) An individual's entire array of single locus genotypes.

Heterozygote — A person who has inherited two different alleles (one from each parent) at a gene locus. Usually interpreted to mean that one of the alleles is expressed normally. See Carrier.

Home brew — Reagents or the combination of reagents made in a laboratory, or purchased reagents used by that laboratory for clinical tests and not for sale to other laboratories.

Homozygote — A person who has inherited identical alleles (one from each parent) at a gene locus.

Locus heterogeneity — Alleles at different gene loci each capable of causing or increasing susceptibility to a disease, for example, alleles at both the BRCA1 and BRCA2 locus can increase susceptibility to breast cancer.

Mendelian — See Single gene (Mendelian) disorder

mRNA — Messenger RNA. The ribonucleic acid (RNA) transcribed from the DNA of a gene in the cell nucleus. mRNA is the template from which proteins are translated.

Metabolite — Usually a low molecular weight compound that is either used in or produced by an enzyme-catalyzed reaction. If the enzyme is dysfunctional, a metabolite used by the reaction it catalyzes will accumulate, whereas a metabolite formed as a result of the reaction will be absent or reduced in concentration.

Mutation — Any change in the nucleotide sequence of DNA.

Nucleotide — The basic unit of DNA, consisting of adenine, cytosine, guanine or thymine, and deoxyribose, and phosphate.

Off label — The use of an FDA-approved drug or device for a purpose other than that intended by the manufacturer and described on the label. FDA only approves drugs or devices for their intended use as described on the label.

Penetrance — The characteristic phenotypic effect of a genotype. If the phenotype is always expressed in the presence of the genotype, the genotype is completely penetrant. If it is not always expressed, it is incompletely penetrant.

Phenotype — The biochemical, physiological, and physical characteristics resulting from the interaction of genotype with environment.

Polymorphism — Frequently occurring variation in a nucleotide sequence. Polymorphisms in genes result in protein polymorphisms. A polymorphism is said to occur when the most common allele has a frequency of no greater than 99%. Some forms of some polymorphisms are associated with increased risk of disease.

Positive predictive value (PPV) — The probability that a person with a positive test result has, or will get, the disease for which the analyte is used as a predictor.

Predisposition test — A test for a genetic predisposition (incompletely penetrant conditions). Not all people with a positive test result will manifest the disease during their lifetimes.

Presymptomatic test — A test for a completely penetrant single-gene disease.

Proficiency testing — The use of blind testing to assess whether the laboratory can perform a test correctly. Usually the samples are provided by an organization independent of the laboratories performing the test.

Protein — String of amino acids linked by peptide bonds. Some proteins have more than one polypeptide chain. Each chain is encoded by a different gene.

Recombinant DNA techniques — The ability to excise exact segments of DNA and insert them into DNA of other organisms, which can then replicate the segment millions of times.

Recessive — A condition that is expressed in homozygotes or in compound heterozygotes (i.e., those who have inherited a different disease-related allele (at the same gene locus) from each parent).

Sensitivity
    Analytical — The probability that a test will detect an analyte when it is present in a specimen.
    Clinical — The probability that a person with a disease, or who will get a disease, will have a positive test result.

Single gene (Mendelian) disorder — The presence of an allele in either single dose (dominant disorders in males or females, X-linked disorders in males), or double dose (recessive disorders), accounts for the presence of disease. The inheritance of these disorders follow the ratios first described by Gregor Mendel.

Somatic mutation — A mutation in the DNA of any cell in the body (somatic cells), except those in the germline.

Specificity
    Analytical — The probability that a test will be negative when an analyte is absent from a specimen.
    Clinical — The probability that a test will be negative in a person free of a disease, and who will not get the disease.

Validity, analytic or clinical — See Positive predictive value, Sensitivity, and Specificity

X-linked — A gene on the X chromosome.

Index

("box" refers to statements or items that appear in the box on the given page)

183

newborn screening, 6, 7, 13, 72, 80, 139; for disorders other than PKU, 147–148; informed consent and, 12–13, 23 box; for sickle cell anemia, 164; state laws, 138
Newborn Screening Quality Assurance Program, CDC, 49n
Nitowsky, H., 142, 147
Nixon, R., 162
non-profit organizations, 104, 126, 128, 130; laboratories of, 8, 9 box, 30 box; 101, 102, 103
nursing, 71–72

Odesina, V., 94
Office for the Protection of Human Subjects from Research Risks, 11 box, 31n, 32, 33, 35
Office of Orphan Products Development, FDA, 77
Office of Rare Diseases, NIH, 11 box, 77, 78, 79, 80, 81, 82, 88
off-label use, 28n, 96
oncology, 106
Oncology Nursing Society, 72n
On-line Mendelian Inheritance in Man (OMIM), 3 box
Oregon, 51
Oregon Health Sciences University, 70n
Orphan Disease Act, 77
osteoporosis, 2
ovarian cancer, 3 box

p-53 gene, 95
parentage testing, 105, 109
Partnership for Genetic Services Pilot Program, 65
patents, 16, 102; and royalties, 16, 112–113
patient rights, 127, 128, 164
Patient Services Department, NORD, 80
Pauling, L., 164
pedigree, 61
peer review, 25, 30
penetrance, 6, 27
Penrose, L., 138
People's Health Council of New York, 164
pharmaceutical industry, 78
phenotype, 6
phenylketonuria (PKU), 1 box, 7, 72, 137–150; dietary management of, 144–146; ferric chlorid test for, 23 box, 139; frequency of, 142; history of, 149; intellectual achievement in,

141; reimbursement for treatment of, 145; screening, history of, 137–144
physicians, knowledge of genetics, 63, 63 box
Physician's Guide to Rare Diseases, (NORD), 79
physicians' office laboratories, 44 box
pilot programs, 27, 43
pneumoccal vaccines, 165
polymerase chain reaction, 23 box
polymorphisms, 1, 2 box, 24, 25, 95
positive predictive value, 26, 27, 31, 95, 130, 161
post-market surveillance, 35
pre-market approval: of genetic tests, 77, 93, 168; conditional, 36, 38, 42
pre-market notification of FDA (Section 510 [k]), 93, 103
prenatal diagnosis, 6, 102, 126, 165, 166
prenatal screening, 6, 72; professional society statements and, 7
Presidential Advisory Commission on Mental Retardation, 139
President's Commission for the Study of Ethical Problems in Medicine and Biomedical and Behavioral Research, 14
presymptomatic tests, 6
pre-test disclosure, 23 box
prevalence of disease, 26
primary care, 70; providers of, 60, 60 box, 61, 62
privacy, 104
professional societies, 8, 10, 38, 87
proficiency testing, 41, 44 box, 48, 97, 98, 103, 115, 116; in hemoglobinopathies, 49; in newborn screening, 49; in prenatal screening, 49, 50 box; publication of results of, 52; sanctions in, 48; in Tay-Sachs screening, 49, 50
profit, 77; and genetic testing, 35, 42n, 115
promotional materials, 93. See also informational materials
prophylactic surgery, 28
proposed recommendations, Task Force on Genetic Testing, 5
prospective studies, 27
psychologists, 29
psychosocial issues, 28, 32 box, 95, 125, 129, 144, 169
psychosocial research, in testing of minors, 13
public education, 5

public health facilities, 62, 72, 73
public knowledge of genetics, 64

quality. See laboratory quality

race and genetics, 163
randomized controlled trial, 27
rare diseases. See diseases, rare
Reagan administration, 168
recontact of subjects, 12, 31, 32 box
referral to a genetics specialist, 62
regulatory issues, 101, 109
Reidy, P.J., 72n
relatives, communication with, 4, 4 box, 68
reliability of tests, 25, 169
repository of cell lines and DNA, 53
residency training, 65, 66, 87
RET oncogene, 96
review. See genetic tests, new, review of
Rhode Island, 140
Rochester, N.Y., 165
Rollins, B., 163
royalties, 16. See also patents

Safe Medical Devices Act of 1990, 77; humanitarian device exemption of, 77, 78
Salas, A., 65
schizophrenia, 24, 141
Schmeck, H. Jr., 140
Schneider, Katherine, 67 box
schools of nursing, 73, 87
schools of public health, 73, 87
schools of social work, 73, 87
Schuett, V., 144
scientific merit of protocols for genetic test development, 31–33; checklist for, 32 box
Scriver, C., 146, 149
Secretary of Health and Human Services, 10, 11, 87
sensitivity. See analytic sensitivity, clinical sensitivity
Seward, P. John, 34n
sex selection, 111
sickle cell anemia, 1 box, 7, 12, 23 box, 77, 148, 162–165; screening for, 72; screening laws, 162; Sickledex test for, 23 box, 163
sickle cell nondisease, 164
single-gene disease. See Mendelian disease
Snow, Karen, 37 box

185

Library of Congress Cataloging-in-Publication Data

Task Force on Genetic Testing (U.S.)
    Promoting safe and effective genetic testing in the United States : final report of the Task Force on
Genetic Testing / edited by Neil A. Holtzman and Michael S. Watson.
        p.   cm.
Includes bibliographical references and index.
ISBN 0-8018-5952-2 (alk. paper).—ISBN 0-8018-5972-7 (pbk : alk. paper)
    1. Human chromosome abnormalities—Diagnosis—Standards—United States.   I. Holtzman,
Neil A. (Neil Anton), 1934–   II. Watson, Michael S.   III. Title.
    RB155.5.T38   1998
    616'.042—dc21   98-16052   CIP